Communication in Elderly Care

Continuum International Publishing Group

The Tower Building
11 York Road
London SE1 7NX

80 Maiden Lane
Suite 704
New York, NY 10038

www.continuumbooks.com

British Library Cataloguing-in-Publication Data
A catalogue record for this book is available from the British Library.

ISBN: 978-1-4411-1254-5 (hardback)

Library of Congress Cataloguing-in-Publication Data
A catalog record for this book is available from the Library of Congress.

Typeset by Newgen Imaging Systems Pvt Ltd, Chennai, India
Printed and bound in Great Britain

Contents

Preface by Nikolas Coupland

Old age, as a concept, is very much a product of its time. We may feel that 60 years is long enough for a person to make a category transition between childhood and old age. It is also long enough, in terms of social change, to have seen postwar economic recoveries and expansion, then deindustrialization and a sharp decline in the prevalence of manual labor, technological advances and transformations in health care science and provision, improvements in welfare provision, the invention of "retirement," and so on. Very clearly these have not been universal or universally progressive shifts; but they are the historical backdrop to most of the national and cultural settings dealt with in this book. The concept of "the elderly," or at least contemporary understandings of what it means to be old, are a rather direct legacy of historically transformed social arrangements and opportunities. At the same time, old age inevitably features in new patterns of intergenerational politics, both formal and informal.

The last 60 years have also seen the strongest-yet wave of globalization. This implies not only demographic mobility (in which many older people have not fully taken part) as well as rampant commodification and consumerism, but also some less tangible shifts. There are good reasons to believe that social being is itself subject to greater commodification, that social identities (for example, not only those linked to nation, class, and gender but also age), which were formally quite consolidated, are nowadays more malleable and uncertain. The life project itself seems more subject to commodified appraisal and negotiation—"what have I achieved, and what is my life worth?" Media reflexively stylize social identities, offering us radically diverse but perhaps equally ungrounded and largely unattainable images of (what the media themselves define as) youth, middle age and the different conditions and types of old age.

No wonder, then, that we see interdisciplinary research nowadays on what it means to be old, and on how societies are coming to terms with increased human longevity on the one hand and shifting ideologies of aging on the other. The sharpest edge of these struggles involves the most vulnerable older people in any given society, and hence the policies and practices of so-called "elderly care." This book makes a welcome contribution to understanding the enactment of care for old people, in its highly diverse national, institutional and interactional contexts, and to developing critical perspectives on it—with an eye to intervention and improvement.

In my own earlier work with colleagues on the sociolinguistics of aging, we initially strove to keep clear of institutional contexts and concerns. We wanted to avoid the assumption that old age is inherently or "naturally" of academic interest only when issues of dependency and care are uppermost. What we found, of course, was that, even in "everyday" contexts of talk, themes of declining health-in-aging, morale, and expectations were far from absent. We managed to locate a set of ideological presuppositions—age-circumscribing and often age-prejudicial discourses—that routinely acted as resources for talk about old age, but also for older people's own talk about themselves. Those discourses continued to be very much at work when we moved from researching everyday exchanges to researching geriatric medical consultations. We argued that the institution of geriatric medicine, at least as it was in evidence in our British data at that time, was engaged in anti-agist ideological campaigning, at the level of policy but also at the level of spoken interaction. The "problems" that patients and practitioners alike were confronting seemed to be as much ideological as biomedical and welfare related.

There are many points of contact between our own earlier studies and those reported in the present volume. It remains important to locate and debate dominant ideologies in the context of elderly care and of aging more generally. Likewise we need to be critically aware of where the boundary between the institutional and the non-institutional lies, and how it is defined. As some contributors to the present book explain, the condition of old age is not inherently decremental and institutionalized care is received by only a minority of older people. Those in care are a highly diverse population and indeed not a single "social group" in any significant sense. Not only do they span some forty plus years of chronological age, they range from the healthy to the seriously ill and from "fully-functioning" (which has always been a worryingly mechanistic attribution) to people with severe cognitive impairment. "Care homes" are themselves enormously diverse, ranging from elite and opulent hotels to disgraceful and demeaning hostels. No wonder that local reactions to institutionalized care for the old can range from abhorrence to deep respect for professional excellence.

The contributions to this book offer many profound insights and positive practical suggestions for care of the elderly with respect to communication and social relations. The two most basic insights for caregivers, through their (sometimes inadequate) training, might be the following. First, the old are not a natural social group. Social histories have generated an age cohort which, in most national settings, is unusually diverse—ranging from the most to the least affluent, the widest to the narrowest of social experiences, the most conservative to the most progressive, and so on. The old include some people for whom modernist postwar structures persisted, and who tend to hold on to a sense of "traditional values," a durable and prescriptive social order. Some others pioneered rock 'n' roll culture, feminism, new ecological sensitivities, mobility and much of the diversity that late modernity has (in patches) tended to foster. The old are in many senses the pioneers of social change and of its legacy in late modernity.

The second insight relates to my use of pronouns like "they" in the preceding paragraph. The old are not "them"; they are "us." It is psychoanalytically understandable that those who progressively age (that is, all of us) should in some ways fear old age and try to sequester it, investing it either with stereotypes of incompetence, misery, and "unwatchability," or alternatively the rosy glow of wisdom and a golden age lifestyle. In contexts of care it is too easy to fall prey to either of these stereotypic constellations, or to some mix of them which is liable to give rise to what is called "elderspeak," which in earlier work we tried to model as under- and over-accommodation by the young to the old. With hindsight, the initial limitation of this perspective was our own willingness to acquiesce to an explicitly "intergroup" model of generational relations, premised on "us and them." In my own case, it was doubtless easier to do this as a "younger researcher" orienting to the sociolinguistics of a late life that I had in view, but did not have in my own personal experience. But my point here is that age-in-years is not the decisive criterion for intergenerationality or for personal identity.

It is tempting to follow Adolf Guggenbühl-Craig's thoughts about old age and the "corruption of myth" and argue that the old are as likely to be "foolish" as wise, as a way of debunking even a favorable stereotyped attribution. There can indeed be damaging implications—indeed a benign agism—in assuming that the old deserve to be accommodated through specific strategies, and not least through strategies of social interaction and language. And this takes us directly into one of the key dilemmas of elderly care. Contributors to this volume eloquently make the case for the centrality of language and communication in delivering what we have to think of as acceptable or successful or appropriate (or, better even, excellent) institutional care. The prior difficulty is in defining those qualitative dimensions. A prescription such as "avoid patronizing talk" has relevance and applicability, especially as research incrementally confirms that residents are regularly subject to what we can reliably characterize as patronizing (or overly accommodative) talk which the residents regularly dislike. On the other hand, the wider "quality" or "excellence" of social interaction that we aspire to will not ultimately be reducible to register choice, which itself presumes that older people in care constitute a single addressee group amenable to a single-style pattern of address. There are more fundamental principles which—difficult as they are to expose and critically examine in training contexts—define the parameters of excellence in communicated care.

The sociolinguistic constitution of care has its basis in the demands and affordances of institutional relations and, as part of those, the multifaceted roles of caregivers and care receivers. To label them that way is already to understate the complexities of those roles, for instance, when a "care home" needs to be a "home" (with the autonomy and security that this connotes) as well as an institution, and when "caregiver" and "care receiver" need to negotiate and transcend the role relationships that these terms imply. As some authors in this collection explain, to give excellent care is sometimes to step outside the regimented and controlling identity of "caregiver," just as the "care receiver" needs, where possible, to facilitate and develop interpersonal rather than role-relevant stances. There will no doubt be occasions where the "foolishness" of an old resident, or a caregiver, is also in the mix, and where interpersonal relations will necessarily reflect this. In research this is where rich understandings of interpersonal alignments, styles, and stances become essential, in the manner of contemporary conversation analysis or interactional sociolinguistics. Studies in this collection dealing with humor, paralinguistic indexicalities and multimodal resources for talk identify important areas for judicious intervention, even though more programmatic research in these and similar fields of elderly care practice is certainly required.

Overall, the volume confirms the importance of a broadly based sociolinguistic research perspective on language and later life, and on language and institutional care as part of that program. I would argue that we need to keep local and global processes in view simultaneously. We need to continue to contextualize research into specific frames and modes of talk with studies of the wider discourses within which local institutional events are contained and legitimized. In the 1980s we were already hearing the rhetoric that "the elderly are coming!" This was a discourse of moral and statistical panic around changes in what demographers call "fertility rates" associated with the baby boomer generation, a swelling old age sector which (the rhetoric implied) would bankrupt societies and drain the working adult sector. This was a classic "them and us" discourse, which made its own contribution to social divisions around age, threatening "society" (a category which of course excluded the old) with the specter of a passive but care-demanding and resource-needy elderly hoard.

We hear that rhetoric today, even more loudly and internationally, spiced up by the global financial crisis. Statistics about aging societies clearly need to be handled with sensitivity, and probably more sensitivity than is currently in evidence. As is often the case, there are real social and economic challenges associated with this particular moral panic in many societies, and the coming decade is likely to see a managed repositioning of boundaries between work and retirement and between midlife and old age. But, as mentioned above, old age will necessarily be reassuringly difficult to pigeonhole and decidedly a matter for us all to renegotiate. It will fall in no small measure to linguists and communication researchers to monitor the developing discourses and their impact, particularly on the minority of older people in need of care.

Cardiff University
September 2010

Introduction

Peter Backhaus

If one thing holds true about old age, it is that it is something that, except by untimely death, no one can "escape." Being old is a potential property of every one of us, irrespective of our current age. Just as today's old were yesterday's youngsters, the newborn baby will be tomorrow's "elderly citizen." It is this inevitability that essentially distinguishes old age from most other features of our identity such as gender, race, class, and culture, definable as they are in relatively stable terms. This makes old age a highly fascinating research topic both for the humanities and for the social sciences.

Recent demographic developments in most postindustrial societies have it that an ever increasing number of old people face an ever decreasing number of young people. In consequence, this means that elderly care is becoming a hot issue across the globe. The present volume looks at this issue from the point of view of language and communication. Studies on this topic so far have been relatively few and far between—scattered through different disciplines such as sociolinguistics, social psychology, speech pathology and aging studies, and their respective publication outputs. The aim of this book is to bring together some of these different types of approaches in one volume.

The contributions to *Communication in Elderly Care* include studies from seven different locations: the United States, Canada, Australia, New Zealand, Denmark, Germany, and Japan. The types of care covered range from informal, noninstitutional networks and semi-institutional arrangements such as home help and migrant-in-the-family systems to assisted living facilities and residential nursing homes.

Kristine Williams starts with an overview of communication problems in institutional care settings in the United States, particularly regarding the frequently and cross-culturally observable use of "elderspeak" by caring staff. Her empirical data provide evidence of the negative effects of this linguistic register on communication in elderly care. This being done, Williams then goes on to report on a brief, in-house training program for caring staff that can be used to minimize the occurrence of elderspeak in institutional care. First tests have shown promising results.

Communication programs for care workers are also the focus of the next two chapters. Boyd Davis and Mary Smith report on a recent staff program intended to improve communication with people suffering from dementia or other cognitive impairments. Working with the Carolinas Conversations Collection, a larger digital database containing both audio and visual recordings of interviews with persons in different stages of dementia, the authors identify four simple rhetorical strategies for nursing staff to substantially improve communication in dementia care.

Drawing on her experiences from over three decades of research in speech pathology, Rosemary Lubinski outlines a tripartite model for creating a more satisfying communicative environment in long-term care settings. Lubinski emphasizes that communication in institutional elderly care can be, and urgently needs to be, improved by taking into account (i) the care receivers' specific communication skills, (ii) strategies that reduce communication breakdowns and facilitate communication for those with physical or cognitive impairments, and (iii) the provision of a more communication friendly environment.

Care of people with Alzheimer's disease in New Zealand is the topic of the next chapter. Margaret Maclagan and Annabel Grant work out the positive effects of reminiscence and the (re)telling of life stories in conversations with dementia patients. Reporting on two long-term studies, the authors demonstrate how skilled conversational partners can help improve the communicative skills of people suffering from dementia despite the cognitive decline that goes hand in hand with the disease.

Trine Heinemann studies interactions between caregivers and care recipients in the Danish home help system. She uses a conversation analytical framework to examine how the relationship between host and home helper becomes increasingly institutionalized, resulting in a serious loss of autonomy of the host and a growing power asymmetry in favor of the helper—a process that is detrimental to the care receiver's independence and sense of dignity.

The next contribution by Hilke Engfer deals with a relatively new type of care arrangement that is getting increasingly popular in Germany as well as other European countries: the migrant-in-the-family model. In this arrangement, an older person is looked after by a foreign care worker cohabiting with that person at his or her place. Using data from a larger case study, this chapter provides an in-depth analysis of a conversation between a Polish live-in and the eldest daughter of a German Alzheimer's patient on the topic of the patient's eating disorders. The analysis reveals that the two interlocutors construe their contributions in different, largely irreconcilable frames. This, Engfer argues, may have negative effects on the quality of the care as a whole.

Differing role relationships between caregivers and care recipients in a Japanese caring facility are the topic of the next chapter. I identify two different modes of talk distinguished by their groundedness in the institutional context. Two examples show how the interlocutors skillfully use these different modes of talk to define and redefine their relationship. I suggest that such flexibility in role relationship construction can have positive effects on the well-being of both caregiver and care recipient.

Yoshiko Matsumoto compares conversations between elderly people inside and outside institutional contexts in Japan. Her focus is on casual conversations that despite their serious content such as illness and death involve much humor and laughter by the participants. She argues that the presentation of grave matter in a mundane, quotidian frame provides an important resource—both in institutional and in private contexts—for regaining an older person's identity.

The next chapter reports on a recent project in Australia in which Alzheimer's patients have been invited to participate in guided museum tours. Heidi Hamilton examines the speech data from these tours with special focus on the effects of different paintings on the patients' communicative behavior. Her study shows that some paintings stimulate communication more easily than others. These findings may be used to design future art programs for individuals with Alzheimer's disease, both in Australia and elsewhere.

The relationship between art and dementia is also in the focus of the final chapter, in which Ellen Ryan and Lori Schindel Martin discuss a variety of narrative techniques that can be used to improve communication in elderly care. The authors show how activities such as storytelling, life writing, and poetry help demented persons to express themselves through verbal art even as the disease proceeds. The authors emphasize that their experiences with using these activities do not show "the stereotypical 'loss of self' but rather ongoing and creative efforts to cope with dementia as a manageable disability".

Communication in Elderly Care contains a great variety of methodologies and approaches, reflecting the differing disciplinary backgrounds and research interests of the contributors. The resulting heterogeneity is no accident, but fully intentional. It serves to remind us that there is no single best way of dealing with the topic, but many possible ways, each of them potentially contributing to our understanding of care communication and what can be done to improve it. Attempts to standardize have been kept to a minimum, which shows most straightforwardly in the different types of transcription systems the authors use to bring their points home.

One underlying feature that unites the different approaches brought together here is their explicitly applied perspective. In order to demonstrate how the authors' research findings can be used in practice, each chapter closes with specific suggestions to care practitioners about how communication in elderly care can be improved. In doing so, we are well aware that it is impossible to provide a ready-made toolkit that fits all circumstances. Indeed, in some cases the authors even suggest contradictory measures, such as the use of open-ended questions for instance, which is recommended by Lubinski but discouraged by Davis and Smith. This goes to show the difficulties about making concrete suggestions in the first place. These difficulties notwithstanding, the contributors to this volume share a belief in the power of language and the way it can change the quality of elderly care.

Acknowledgments

We gratefully acknowledge a grant from the Fritz Thyssen Foundation, a Waseda University Grant for Special Research Projects (Project No.2010A-835), as well as the generous financial and personal support from the German Institute for Japanese Studies Tokyo. Many thanks to Stanislaw Eberlein for his invaluable editing support.

This book is dedicated to Helene Mehl (1915–1997).

Chapter 1

Elderspeak in Institutional Care for Older Adults

Kristine N. Williams

Introduction

Communication is of critical importance to residents of elder care institutions, such as nursing homes, as a means to maintain both a connection with other persons and a sense of self (Buron 2008). The importance of social relationships is described in Maslow's hierarchy of needs which places the human need for affiliation second only to survival and safety (Maslow 1954). "Successful aging" is defined not only as physical and functional health, but also as high cognitive functioning and involvement with society (Rowe and Kahn 1997). Active engagement with others through productive activity and interpersonal relationships is necessary to realize functional capacities and achieve successful aging.

Nursing home (NH) communication has long been characterized as insufficient in both quantity and quality by residents and social scientists alike (Buron 2008; Grau et al. 1995; Lubinski 1995; Nussbaum 1991). Research has demonstrated that limited staff-resident communication focuses on care tasks instead of personal concerns, is controlling, and ultimately encourages dependency (Baltes and Wahl 1996; Carpiac-Claver and Levy-Storms 2007; Grainger 1995; Iwasiw and Olson 1995; Levy-Storms 2008; Williams et al. 2005). Correspondingly, NH residents who engage in interpersonal communication and relationships with staff tend to live longer (Kiely et al. 2000), and residents themselves report that communication with staff is an aspect of care that is highly valued (Grau et al. 1995).

Research has established that communication training for NH staff improves institutional communication (Levy-Storms 2008; Williams et al. 2003; Williams 2006). McGilton and colleagues (2003) report that such training increases positive interactions and results in relationship-promoting communication during care, whereas Burgio and colleagues (2002) have documented increased positive statements from certified nursing assistants after training as well as reductions in ineffective communication. NH residents themselves have reported improved staff nonverbal communication and increased personal (versus task-focused) messages after the staff underwent communication training (Medvene et al. 2006; van Weert et al. 2005).

Quality of care, it has been shown, also increases after NH staff communication training (Levy-Storms 2008). Other studies report that NH residents even experienced reduced anxiety and increased satisfaction with care after staff training and that staff stress was also reduced (Finnema et al. 2005; Grosch et al. 2008). Furthermore, staff use of individualized communication care plans succeeded not only in increasing resident engagement in sustained and meaningful conversations with staff (Acton et al. 2007), the training has also reduced agitation and other problem behaviors in residents with dementia (Burgio et al. 2002; McCallion et al. 1999; Roth et al. 2002).

One prevalent and problematic speech style used by NH staff is called elderspeak. Elderspeak is a common intergenerational speech style used by younger persons in communication with older adults in a variety of community and health care settings. Based on negative stereotypes of older adults as less competent communicators, younger speakers (in this case NH staff) modify their communication with NH residents by simplifying the vocabulary and grammar and by adding clarifications such as repetitions and altered prosody, resulting in changes in affective messages within dimensions of care, respect, and control. Intended to show a caring attitude and improve communication, staff elderspeak communication actually sounds like baby-talk and may lead to negative outcomes. This paper provides an overview of the current knowledge of elderspeak, its characteristics and prevalence across institutional care settings in the United States, and the negative outcomes associated with elderspeak use by NH staff. It starts with a brief general overview of institutional care for older adults in the United States and will demonstrate why staff training to overcome elderspeak is an effective means to improve the quality of NH care.

Institutional Care for Older Adults in the United States

The population of older adults continues to grow in the United States and reflects the expansion of the aging population in other developed countries and around the world. The number of persons over 65 years of age increased by 13% from 1998 to 2008, growing by 4.5 million to reach 38.9 million. Currently, one in eight U.S. citizens is 65 years of age or older. As life expectancy continues to increase, the older adult population is projected to increase from 40 million in 2010 to 55 million by 2020, a 36% increase (Administration on Aging 2010).

In 2008, approximately 1.6 million (4.1%) of older Americans lived in institutional care settings where they needed support in performing activities of daily living (ADLs): bathing, using the toilet, dressing, eating, etc. The majority (1.4 million) of these individuals resided in NH facilities. The typical resident of a NH in the United States requires assistance with 3.75 ADLs (Lawton and Brody 1969; NCAL 2001). Alternative residential care facilities developed more recently include assisted living that serves older adults who need lower levels of support. Assisted living currently serves approximately 1 million older adults, a population expected to double in the next decade (Mollica and Johnson-Lemarche 2005; NCAL 2007). Other senior citizen housing options include congregate senior apartments that serve approximately 2.4% of older adults and provide at least one supportive service such as meals (Administration on Aging 2010).

Care for older adults in NHs and other facilities is institutionally regimented and results in a loss of control and autonomy when making everyday decisions (Gubrium 1975; Hayley et al. 1996). In addition, traditional health care provider-patient relationships reflect an imbalance of power in which older adults assume the sick role. Most NH residents are primarily cared for by certified nursing assistants. These paraprofessionals have limited education and training in elderly care, especially in meeting psychosocial needs. Many come from educational and socio-economic backgrounds that are different from those of nursing home residents. Staffing shortages and high turnover rates make work in a NH physically and emotionally demanding and stressful (Cohen-Mansfield 1995). Changes in federal and state licensure regulations have been enacted to improve the quality of NH care prompting a culture change that has been adopted to make NH care more resident-centered and less task-oriented and institutional (White et al. 2008). Training staff to reduce elderspeak is one approach to improve staff-resident communication.

Elderspeak

Elderspeak is a speech style commonly used by younger adults interacting with older adults and occurs across societies and cultures (Backhaus 2009; de Bot and Makoni 2005; Grainger 1993; Kihlgren et al. 1994). Elderspeak, or "secondary baby talk," was first characterized by Caporael (1981), who found that it made up 20% of staff-resident interactions in NHs. She identified the slower speaking rate, exaggerated intonation, elevated pitch and volume, greater repetition, simpler vocabulary, and reduced grammatical complexity as being typical of elderspeak. Another aspect of intergenerational speech common to institutions is overly directive or overbearing talk, frequently referred to as patronizing speech (Ryan et al. 1991). Both overly directive and overly nurturing communication occur frequently as forms of elderspeak and may negatively influence the lives of older adults residing in NHs. Characteristic features of elderspeak include over-simplification and clarification strategies and alterations in emotional tone, and they all imply incompetence on the part of the listener (Ryan, Hummert and Boich 1995). Simplification of syntax includes reductions in the length of sentences, number of embedded verb clauses, and grammatical complexity and is reflected in both the vocabulary used by a younger person or care staff member and the density of the ideas communicated to an older adult. Repetitions and altered prosody are attempts to clarify speech. This includes paraphrasing or word-for-word repetition of communication content as well as the high pitch and intonation characteristics of " 'baby talk."

Other characteristic features of elderspeak include the use of diminutives, tag questions, and collective pronouns. Diminutives include terms of endearment such as "good girl," "honey," and "dear" and imply parent-child dynamics. The use of collective pronouns when the singular form is grammatically correct implies that the older adult cannot act alone. For example, "Do we want to go back to our room now?" Tag questions, such as "You want to get dressed now, don't you?" appear to offer a choice to the listener. However, the implication is that the speaker had to guide the listener to select the appropriate response. These characteristic features of elderspeak all imply indirectly that the listener is incompetent and dependent.

Other significant characteristics of elderspeak are modifications in nonverbal communication such as prosody, gaze, facial expression, proximity, and gestures (Ryan et al.1994). They too significantly alter the underlying emotional or affective messages in communication within dimensions of care, respect, and control. In fact, nursing staff may add diminutives (terms of endearment) and other verbal and nonverbal features of elderspeak to soften the underlying messages of control typical in institutional care; the message itself varies depending on the words (and voice tone and other nonverbal behaviors). For example, the controlling message "You need to get in your room [pointing]" may be softened by elderspeak as follows: "Come on *honey* [diminutive], *we*'ll [collective versus individual pronoun] find *our* [collective pronoun] room down by the *potty* [childish reference]." The overly caring tone overcomes the message of control. However, this results in an overly nurturing, infantilizing message.

Alteration in emotional tone is a qualitative aspect of elderspeak that reflects an imbalance of care and control (Hummert and Ryan 1996). Normal adult speech exemplifies affirming emotional tone, indicating that the older adult is competent to comprehend the message and act independently. In contrast, elderspeak implies a lack of competence on behalf of the listener, requiring the speaker to assist or direct the conversational partner. Patronizing messages can be classified as overly nurturing, reflecting high care and low control, or directive, reflecting a high degree of control and little caring (Hummert et al. 1998).

The following is a transcript of a typical conversation illustrating the modified communication of elderspeak. It was recorded during a research study in which a NH certified nurse assistant speaks with a resident during morning care (Williams 2001). This example includes simplified vocabulary and childish reference to the resident:

> Jenny... Where's your legs?... Hangin' off the bed girl... hanging off the bed... Hey Jenny... You're zonked this morning aren't ya girlie?...... Sound asleep.

The Communication Predicament of Aging

Communication Accommodation Theory (Giles et al. 1991) describes how conversational partners modify speech during social interactions. Participants in conversation universally accommodate, or modify, their speech and language in order to match or minimize differences with the person with whom they are communicating. Accommodation has been observed in a variety of populations including persons of differing native tongues as well as intergenerational dyads. Over- and under-accommodation occur when one person misunderstands the needs of the communication partner or alters communication purposefully for therapeutic goals. For older adults, consequences of positive accommodation are important in achieving social support and in receiving information that they can comprehend from medical practitioners. However, over-accommodation may encourage dependent behavior and the assumption of the role of a patient.

The Communication Predicament of Aging Model (Ryan et al. 1986) applies Communication Accommodation Theory specifically to the world of older adults. In this model, the younger communication partner recognizes visual or other clues as to the advanced age of the conversational partner. This triggers stereotypical ideas about older adults as a group being less competent communicators (Hummert et al. 1994). In addition, older adults are perceived to have sharply declining abilities, dependency needs, and a desire to disengage. Because of these stereotypes, of which the younger adult may not be aware, younger partners alter their speech to meet the assumed needs of the older person. Alterations may include limiting content to safe topics, speaking louder and in shorter sentences, using simplistic vocabulary, as well as emphasizing and repeating key words.

The older adult receiving this message may recognize these changes and may adopt a self-concept consistent with his or her own negative stereotype of older adults, thus enacting a self-fulfilling prophecy of being old and feeling old. In order to avoid further reminders of this negative identity, older adults may avoid interacting with younger adults who provide these messages. Repeated exposure to elderspeak may contribute to decreased self-esteem and depression, withdrawal from further social encounters, and the assumption of behaviors consistent with negative stereotypes of aging (Rodin and Langer 1980). This predicament is part of a negative feedback loop that affects future communication encounters. Persons with obvious physical or cognitive disabilities frequently receive patronizing talk (Hummert 1994; Kemper et al. 1998), and those in environments suggesting dependency, such as in institutions, trigger more speech accommodations than older adults in community settings (Hummert et al. 1998). If persons outside the communication dyad observe a patronizing interaction, they may assume that the older adult benefits from the accommodations. In their future interactions with that older person, they may accordingly employ elderspeak. In effect, elderspeak is thus reinforced, and the recipient of elderspeak may, in the worst cases, even be blamed for its occurrence.

From an interpersonal perspective, elderspeak fails to acknowledge the older adult as an independent actor and indicates that he or she is not a worthy communication partner. Specifically, the metamessage may reflect: (i) "indifference"—that is, denying the existence of the partner; (ii) "imperviousness"—that is, denying the validity of the partner's experiences; or (iii) "disqualification"—that is, denying the significance of the other (Cissna and Siebert 1981). The relational message in elderspeak may insult the self-concept of the older adult.

The communication enhancement model (Ryan, Meredith, et al. 1995) provides a guide for appropriate communication that modifies speech as needed while avoiding over-accommodations. Prior to employing speech modifications, an individual assessment is made of the older adults' communication abilities and limitations. Only accommodations determined necessary to achieve successful staff-resident communication are employed and abilities of the individual older adult are reinforced. For example, limiting complex and abstract sentences may be needed to overcome language and cognitive changes in persons with dementia. Although both positive and negative effects of elderspeak have been explored, further research is needed to determine how best to assess communication needs and to identify speech accommodations to meet individual needs.

Negative Effects of Elderspeak

Cognitively intact older adults readily recognize elderspeak and report negative reactions to this speech style (Kemper and Harden 1999; Leland 7 October 2008). In Kemper and Harden's study, older adults who received spoken directions on how to complete a task from young adults who used elderspeak rated the communication as patronizing and demeaning. They reported more difficulty comprehending instructions and showed no greater accuracy in completing the task than older adults directed by elderspeak-free communication. However, semantic elaboration, including repetitions, paraphrasing, and limiting syntactic complexity, was found to provide some benefits for comprehension. Although elderspeak may be intended to promote effective communication and show caring, research demonstrates that it fails to accomplish these goals (Kemper and Harden 1999).

Relinquishing self-care activities may occur because of depression or as the older individual adopts behaviors consistent with the stereotype of an older adult. Adaptive physiologic reserves are reduced in aging individuals so that reductions in self-care activities requiring motor skills, such as dressing oneself, can lead to a rapid loss of muscle strength, flexibility, and aerobic capacity. This can contribute to a progressive decline in functional status and lead to permanent dependence on others when performing these activities or, in other cases, necessitate a prolonged rehabilitation (Abrams et al. 1995).

Cognitive function is also a " 'use it or lose it" phenomenon. Cognitive theorists postulate that mental exercise promotes optimal cognitive functioning in old age (Salthouse 1999), and evidence suggests that a lack of early or recent cognitive challenge predisposes a decline (Snowdon et al. 1996). Cognitive decline may occur when residents receive simplified communication, characteristic of elderspeak, as opposed to the confirmative and stimulating communication of adult-to-adult encounters. Self-efficacy, or a person's belief in their ability to take appropriate actions (Bandura 1995), has also been associated with the maintenance of cognitive abilities in old age (Lachman and Leff 1989; Lachman et al. 1992). Patronizing communication in the NH encourages residents to be dependent on staff and reduces their self-determination; as a lack of ability or training on the part of the staff, such communication fails to support the self-efficacy of residents and the maintenance of their cognitive skills. Inappropriate speech accommodations may even result in the residents' learned helplessness, an attitude that has been identified as a critical factor in the negative cycle of the Communication Predicament of Aging Model (Rodin and Langer 1980). Messages suggesting incompetence and dependence along with perceived loss of personal control over the environment may result in a passive resident who accepts the care provided but has no motivation or confidence in his or her abilities to think or act independently. This attitude of learned helplessness and lack of self-efficacy may contribute to further declines in cognitive and functional capacities.

Research suggests that some frail and debilitated older adults may derive support and succor from overly nurturing talk and perceive it positively (O'Connor and Rigby 1996). However, elderspeak is perceived negatively by most older adults. Responses to patronizing messages may indirectly contribute to declines in cognition and physical health for older adults who are already frail and infirm. Health care workers who use elderspeak with older adults believe that it improves communication effectiveness and demonstrates caring (Williams and Warren 2009). These well-meaning workers fail to realize the negative messages of elderspeak. However, research has demonstrated that cognitively intact older adults recognize elderspeak communication, find it patronizing, and fail to demonstrate increased comprehension of communication when elderspeak is used (Kemper and Harden 1999). Training staff to enable them to tailor their communication to meet the individually determined needs of care recipients will improve the quality of NH care.

Research Characterizing Elderspeak

Audio recordings of staff-resident communication collected during a series of research studies in nine NHs in the Midwestern United States (Williams 2001; Williams et al. 2003; Williams 2006) document the use of elderspeak in NH communication. Following informed consent to protect the rights of human subjects, three to five recordings of each certified nurse assistant volunteer communicating with different residents during routine care were collected with wireless recording devices. Analysis of the transcribed and psycholinguistically coded transcripts from these three studies indicates consistent staff use of diminutives, that is, inappropriately intimate terms of endearment (M = 5.1 per 100 utterances), as well as the use of the collective "'we" pronoun substitution (M = 5.2 per 100 utterances). Other common features of elderspeak including altered prosody and tag questions were also found.

Although individual certified nurse assistants varied in their use of elderspeak, it was a common communication phenomenon. The frequency of the use of diminutives ranged from 0 to 47 times per 100 utterances, while collective pronoun substitutions occurred at frequencies ranging from 0 to 32 per 100 utterances. A group of naïve judges were asked to rate the recordings of NH staff-resident communication and they found it to be overly nurturing, highly controlling, and less respectful than communication between staff peers.

In order to determine which factors (i.e., nursing home, staff, resident) influence staff use of elderspeak, a reanalysis of 212 recorded caregiving interactions between 50 nursing assistants and residents, representing the nine different NHs in the 2001, 2003, and 2006 studies, was performed (Williams 2005). Analyses of variance of tabulations from transcribed conversations coded for occurrences of elderspeak (diminutives, collective pronoun substitutions, and shortened mean length of utterances) confirmed that individual staff differ in their use of elderspeak communication. Facility variations were also significant.

Factors entered into regression equations to identify predictors of elderspeak were: facility location, size, and ownership of the NH; staff age, gender, experience, and tenure in the facility; as well as resident gender, dementia diagnosis, and functional status. Diminutive use occurred more frequently in urban and rural facilities compared with suburban nursing home facilities. Collective "we" pronoun substitutions were more prevalent in rural and suburban facilities and with residents who were more disabled. Abbreviated sentences were predicted by urban location, smaller facility size, nonprofit NH ownership, and increased staff experience. Differences in the use of elderspeak by nursing staff in each NH facility suggest that speech style may be a part of each NH's culture (Williams 2005).

Elderspeak also extends to assisted living facilities where more limited support is provided for older adults who maintain independent apartments. Although residents of assisted living facilities are younger and healthier than those in nursing homes, care staff still use elderspeak in daily care activities. Assisted living residents identify elderspeak as common and problematic when asked what aspects of life in assisted living they would change. One resident reported: "It's like they think we're children... at least they give the attitude. So I think they should recognize people here are elderly but we aren't stupid and they shouldn't talk to us like we're 3 years old" (quoted in Williams and Warren 2009).

Elderspeak is also prevalent in dementia care institutions. Our research (Williams et al. 2003) found that staff communication with residents suffering from dementia differed from communication with residents without cognitive impairment. Nursing staff increased their use of elderspeak when conversing with residents diagnosed with dementia compared with cognitively intact residents. Significant reductions in the mean length of utterances occurred in talk with residents with dementia, with trends toward reductions in the complexity of vocabulary (type token ratio) and increased collective pronoun substitutions. Thus, elderspeak communication is prevalent and more concentrated in dementia care.

Researchers are beginning to examine specific outcomes of elderspeak communication. In a recent observational study of NH residents with moderate dementia, disruptive behavior referred to as "resistiveness to care" was more than twice as common when nursing care staff used elderspeak compared with normal adult-to-adult communication or when care was conducted in silence (Williams, Herman et al. 2009). Elderspeak communication may fail to meet the communication needs and preferences of persons with dementia who may react with challenging behavior (Algase et al. 1996). In the study by Williams and colleagues, some but not all subjects appeared to be sensitive to elderspeak communication, as reflected in aggressive behaviors and evidence of displeasure.

Outcomes of Elderspeak: Dementia Care

Implicit messages of elderspeak may be especially threatening to the maintenance of self-concept and personhood which is critical to the well-being of persons with dementia (Kitwood 1997; Kitwood and Bredin, 1992). In the United States, as in other countries, the population of persons with dementia who require institutional care is expanding (Alzheimer's Disease International 2009). More than 50% of NH residents and up to two-thirds of assisted living residents have Alzheimer's disease or other dementias (Alzheimer's Association 2008; Hyde et al. 2007).

The struggle to maintain one's personhood remains a critical task for persons with dementia (Kitwood 1997; Kitwood and Bredin 1992; Sabat et al. 2004). Even persons with advanced dementia demonstrate that they maintain a sense of personhood by communicating disagreement through nonverbal behaviors. Thus they continue to be aware of their personal needs and vehemently resist violations of their personal desires and goals (Small et al. 1998). Persons with dementia may communicate their displeasure with patronizing communication through "problem" behaviors such as aggression or resistiveness to care. These behavioral responses may in turn increase the time required to complete care tasks and increase stress for nurses and other care providers who may fear harm or experience actual injuries (Lyman 1993; Novak and Chappell 1996). Nonetheless, some experts advise that elderspeak may positively affect persons with dementia. Sloane and colleagues (1995), for example, advocate staff use of familial forms of address such as "papa" to comfort persons with dementia, whereas Small and colleagues (2000) found that family caregiver's use of collective pronouns was effective in gaining the dementia patient's cooperation with caregiving. However, the ongoing controversy about elderspeak indicates a need for clinical testing.

In an observational study we therefore tested the responses of NH residents with dementia to different types of staff speech including elderspeak communication (Williams et al. 2009). Videotaped care episodes (n = 80) of NH residents with dementia (n = 20) were coded for all types of staff communication (i.e., normal talk, silence, and elderspeak) and subsequent resident behavior (i.e., cooperative versus resistive to care). Through Bayesian statistical analysis we then tested the temporal relationships between staff communication and subsequent resident resistiveness to care. The probability of resistiveness varied significantly with communication, and resistiveness to care behaviors doubled when nursing staff used elderspeak communication as compared with normal talk (Williams et al. 2009). Further research evaluating the underlying affective messages of elderspeak communication determined that messages strongly conveying control were also significantly correlated with resistive behaviors (Williams and Herman, in press). This observational research suggests that negative effects of elderspeak extend to dementia care.

Future Directions: Staff Training to Overcome Elderspeak

Training nursing care staff to minimize or overcome their use of elderspeak communication is promising. A three-session in-service program designed to overcome elderspeak has proven effective in minimizing elderspeak use as determined in audio recordings of daily care with maintained effects over two months (see Williams 2006). The focus of the training was on making nursing staff aware of their use of elderspeak communication and how it may provide negative messages to older adults, as well as teaching effective communication strategies to replace elderspeak. This brief (three one-hour sessions) communication training intervention was well accepted in multiple NH settings where it resulted in significant reductions in elderspeak use with effect sizes (Williams, et al., 2003; Williams, 2006).

As a result of this training program, nursing staff communication also became more person-centered and less task-focused, as a result of which nursing home residents increased their participation in conversations with nursing staff by 5% (Williams et al., 2005). Training has been effective in a total of nine different NH facilities, primarily working with paraprofessional staff or nursing assistants who provide most of the direct care and opportunities for communication for older adult residents. Considering the link between elderspeak communication and resistiveness to care, further research is needed to test the effect of NH staff communication training on resident behavioral outcomes as well as on benefits to staff who may realize greater job satisfaction and lower turnover rates. Improvements in the care and quality of life for older adults may be realized by training staff in more effective communication with older adult care recipients.

Practical Implications

Communication is part of the "art of caring." As health care technologies and work demands increase, health care workers need to remember the importance of communication in caring for older adults and the impact it can have on them psychologically. Communication can be patronizing, even if it is not intended to be. Underlying patronizing messages can have negative effects on older adults. Therefore, health care workers need to be aware of their communication style with older adults and learn how to self-monitor it, as this will effectively improve not only their communication with them, but also the effectiveness of care in institutional care facilities. The research evidence demonstrates that training staff in effective communication skills for working with older adults is one way to improve the quality of care and quality of life in institutional care for older adults.

References

Abrams, W., M. Beers & R. Berkow (eds). (1995). *The Merck Manual of Geriatrics*, 2nd edn Whitehouse Station, NJ: Merck Research Laboratories.

Acton, G. J., S. Yauk, B. A. Hopkins, & P. A. Mayhew. (2007). Increasing social communication in persons with dementia. *Research and Theory in Nursing Practice* 21 (1) 32–44.

Administration on Aging (2010). *A Profile of Older Americans 2009*. www.aoa.gov/AoARoot/Aging_Statistics/Profile/2009/docs/2009profile_508.pdf (accessed 1 April 2010).

Algase, D. L., C. Beck, A. Kolanowski, S. Berrent, K. Richards & E. Beattie. (1996). Need-driven dementia-compromised behavior: An alternative view of disruptive behavior. *American Journal of Alzheimer's Disease and Other Dementias* 11(6) 10–19.

Alzheimer's Association (2008). *Alzheimer's Disease Facts and Figures*. www.alz.org/national/documents/report_alzfactsfigures2008.pdf (accessed April 2008).

Alzheimer's Disease International (2009). *World Alzheimer's Report, 2009*. www.alz.co.uk/research/files/World%20Alzheimer%20Report%20Executive%20Summary.pdf (accessed 6 April 2010).

Backhaus, P. (2009). Politeness in institutional elderly in Japan: A cross-cultural comparison. *Journal of Politeness Research* (5). 53–71.

Baltes, M. M. & H. W. Wahl. (1996). Patterns of communication in old age: The dependence-support and independence-ignore script. *Health Communication* 8 (3). 217–31.

Bandura, A. (1995). *Self-efficacy in Changing Societies*. New York: Cambridge University Press.

Burgio, L., A. Stevens, K. Burgio, D. Roth, P. Paul, & J. Gerstle. (2002). Teaching and maintaining behavior management skills in the nursing home. *The Gerontologist* 42 (4). 487–96.

Buron, B. (2008). Levels of personhood: A model for dementia care. *Geriatric Nursing* 29 (5). 324–32.

Caporael, L. (1981). The paralanguage of caregiving: Baby talk to the institutionalized aged. *Journal of Personality and Social Psychology* 40(5). 876–84.

Carpiac-Claver, M. L. & L. Levy-Storms. (2007). In a manner of speaking: Communication between nurse aides and older adults in long-term care settings. *Health Communication* 22(1). 59–67.

Cissna, K., & Sieberg, E.(1981). Patterns of interactional confirmation and disconfirmation. In C. Wilder-Mott & J. H. Weakland (Eds), *Rigor and Imagination: Essays form the Legacy of Gregory Bateson* (pp. 253–82). New York: Praeger Publishers.

Cohen-Mansfield, J. (1995). Stress in nursing home staff: A review and a theoretical model. *Journal of Applied Gerontology* 14(4). 444–66.

de Bot, K. & S. Makoni. (2005). *Language and Aging in Multilingual Contexts*. Toronto: Multilingual Matters LTD.

Finnema, E., R. Dröes, T. Ettema, M. Ooms, H. Adèr, M. Ribbe & W. van Tilburg (2005). The effect of integrated emotion-oriented care versus usual care on elderly persons with dementia in the nursing home and on nursing assistants: A randomized clinical trial. *International Journal of Geriatric Psychiatry* 20. 330–43.

Giles, H., N. Coupland & J. Coupland. (1991). Accommodation theory: Communication, context, and consequence. In H. Giles, N. Couplan & J. Coupland (eds), *Contexts of Accommodation. Developments in Applied Sociolinguistics*, 1–68. Cambridge: Cambridge University Press.

Grainger, K. (1993). 'That's a lovely bath dear': Reality construction in the discourse of elderly care. *Journal of Aging Studies* 7(3). 247–62.

—(1995). Communication and the institutionalized elderly. In J. F. Nussbaum & J. Coupland (eds), *Handbook of Communication and Aging Research*, 417–36. Mahwah, NJ: Lawrence Erlbaum Associates.

Grau, L., B. Chandler & C. Saunders. (1995). Nursing home residents' perceptions of the quality of their care. *Journal of Psychosocial Nursing* 33(5). 34–41.

Grosch, K., L. Medvene & H. Wolcott (2008). Person-centered caregiving instruction for geriatric nursing assistant students: Development and evaluation. *Journal of Gerontological Nursing* 34(8). 28–31.

Gubrium, J. F. (1975). *Living and Dying at Murray Manor.* New York: St. Martin's Press.

Hayley, D. C., Cassel, C. K., Snyder, L., & Rudberg, M. A. (1996). Ethical and legal issues in nursing home care. *Archives of Internal Medicine, 156,* 249–56.

Hummert, M. L. (1994). Stereotypes of the elderly and patronizing speech. In J. M. Wiemann & J. F. Nussbaum (eds), *Interpersonal Communication in Older Adulthood: Interdisciplinary Research,* 168–89. Newbury Park, CA: Sage.

Hummert, M. L., Garstka, T., Shaner, J., & Strahm, S. (1994). Stereotypes of the Elderly Held by Young, Middle-Aged , and Elderly Adults. *Journal of Gerontology: Psychological Sciences, 49*(5), 240–9.

Hummert, M. L. & E. B. Ryan (1996). Toward understanding variations in patronizing talk addressed to older adults: Psycholinguistic features of care and control. *International Journal of Psycholinguistics* 12(2). 149–69.

Hummert, M. L., J. Shaner, T. Garstka & C. Henry. (1998). Communication with older adults: The influence of age stereotypes, context, and communicator age. *Human Communication Research* 25(1). 124–51.

Hyde, J., R. Perez & B. Forester. (2007). Dementia and assisted living. *The Gerontologist* 47 (Suppl I). 51–67.

Iwasiw, C. L., & J. K. Olson. (1995). Content analysis of non-professional caregiver-patient interactions in long-term care facilities. *Clinical Nursing Research* 4(4). 411–24.

Kemper, S., A. Finter-Urczyk, P. Ferrell, T. Harden & C. Billington. (1998). Using elderspeak with older adults. *Discourse Processes* 25(1). 55–73.

Kemper, S. & T. Harden. (1999). Experimentally disentangling what's beneficial about elderspeak from what's not. *Psychology and Aging* 14(4). 656–70.

Kiely, D. K., M. A. Simon, R. N. Jones & J. N. Morris. (2000). The protective effect of social engagement on mortality in long-term care. *Journal of the American Geriatrics Society* 48(12). 1367–72.

Kihlgren, M., A. Hallgren, A. Norberg & I. Karlsson. (1994). Integrity promoting care of demented patients: Patterns of interaction during morning care. *International Journal of Aging and Human Development* 39(4). 303–19.

Kitwood, T. (1997). The experience of dementia. *Aging and Mental Health* 7. 15–22.

Kitwood, T. & K. Bredin. (1992). Towards a theory of dementia care: Personhood and wellbeing. *Aging and Society* 12. 269–87.

Lachman, M. E. & R. Leff. (1989). Perceived control and intellectual functioning in the elderly. *Psychology and Aging* 2. 266–71.

Lachman, M. E., S. L. Weaver & M. M. Bandura. (1992). Improving memory and control beliefs through cognitive restructuring and self-generated strategies. *Journal of Gerontology: Psychological Sciences* 47. 293–399.

Lawton, M. P. & E. M. Brody. (1969). Assessment of older people: Self-maintaining and instrumental activities of daily living. *Gerontologist* 9. 179–85.

Leland, John. 7 October (2008). In 'Sweetie' and 'Dear', a hurt beyond insult for the elderly. *The New York Times.* www.nytimes.com/2008/10/07/us/07aging.html (last accessed 8 September 2010).

Levy-Storms, L. (2008). Therapeutic communication training in long-term care institutions: Recommendations for future research. *Patient Education and Counseling* 73. 8–21.

Lubinski, R. (1995). State-of-the-art perspectives on communication in nursing homes. *Topics in Language Disorders* 15(2). 1–19.

Lyman, K. (1993). *Day in, Day Out with Alzheimer's: Stress in Caregiving Relationships.* Philadelphia: Temple University Press.

Maslow, A. H. (1954). *Motivation and Personality.* New York: Harper and Row.

McCallion, P., R. Toseland, D. Lacey & S. Banks. (1999). Educating nursing assistants to communicate more effectively with nursing home residents. *The Gerontologist* 39(5). 546–58.

McGilton, K. S, L. L. O'Brien-Pallas, G. Darlington, M. Evans, F. Wynn & D. M. Pringle. (2003). Effects of a relationship-enhancing program of care on outcomes. *Journal of Nursing Scholarship* 35(2). 151–6.

Medvene, L., K. Grosch & N. Swink. (2006). Interpersonal complexity: A cognitive component of person-centered care. *The Gerontologist* 46. 220–6.

Mollica, R. & H. Johnson-Lemarche. (2005). State residential care and Assisted living policy: 2004. http://aspe.hhs.gov/daltcp/reports/04alcom.htm. (accessed 24 May 2007).

NCAL (National Center for Assisted Living). (2001). *Assisted Living: Independence, Choice, and Dignity.* www.ncal.org/about/alicd.pdf (accessed 30 June 2008).

—,(2007). *Assisted Living Resident Profile.* Retrieved May 24, 2007, from www.ncal.org/about/resident.cfm.

Novak, M. & N. L. Chappell. (1996). The impact of cognitively impaired patients and shift on nursing assistant stress. *International Journal of Aging and Human Development* 43(3). 235–48.

Nussbaum, J. F. (1991). Communication, language and the institutionalised elderly. *Aging and Society* (11). 149–65.

O'Connor, B. & H. Rigby. (1996). Perceptions of baby talk, frequency of receiving baby talk, and self-esteem among community and nursing home residents. *Psychology and Aging* 11(1). 147–54.

Rodin, J. & E. J. Langer. (1980). Aging labels: The decline of control and the fall of self-esteem. *Journal of Social Issues* 36. 12–29.

Roth, D. L., A. B. Stevens, L. D. Burgio & K. L. Burgio. (2002). Timed-event sequential analysis of agitation in nursing home residents during personal care interactions with nursing assistants. *Journals of Gerontology Series B-Psychological Sciences & Social Sciences* 57(B). 461–8.

Rowe, J. W. & R. L. Kahn, R. L. (1997). Successful aging. *The Gerontologist* 37. 433–40.

Ryan, E. B., R. Y. Bourhis & U. Knops. (1991). Evaluative perceptions of patronizing speech addressed to elders. *Psychology and Aging* 6(3). 442–50.

Ryan, E. B., H. Giles, R. Y. Bartolucci & K. Henwood. (1986). Psycholinguistic and social psychological components of communication by and with the elderly. *Language and Communication* 6(1/2). 1–24.

Ryan, E. B., M. L. Hummert & L. H. Boich. (1995). Communication predicaments of aging: Patronizing behavior toward older adults. *Journal of Language and Social Psychology* 14(1–2). 144–66.

Ryan, E. B., M. Maclean & J. B. Orange. (1994). Inappropriate accommodation in communication to elders: Inferences about nonverbal correlates. *International Journal of Aging and Human Development* 39(4). 273–91.

Ryan, E. B., S. D. Meredith, M. J. MacLean & J. B. Orange. (1995). Changing the way we talk with elders: Promoting health using the communication enhancement model. *International Journal of Aging and Human Development* 41. 89–107.

Sabat, S., L. Napolitano & H. Fath. (2004). Barriers to the construction of a valued social identity: A case study of Alzheimer's disease. *American Journal of Alzheimer's Disease and Other Dementias* 19. 177–85.

Salthouse, T. (1999). Theories of cognition. In V. L. Bengtson & K. W. Schaie (eds), *Handbook of Theories of Aging,* 196–208. New York: Springer Publishing Company.

Sloane, P., V. J. Honn, S. A. R. Dwyer, J. Weiselquist, C. Cain & S. Meyers. (1995). Bathing the Alzheimer's patient in long-term care: Results and recommendations from three studies. *American Journal of Alzheimer's Disease and Other Dementias* 10(4). 3–11.

Small, J., K. Geldart, Gutman, G., & Scott, M. A. (1998). The discourse of self in dementia. *Ageing and Society, 18,* 291–316.

Small, J., Geldart, K., & G. Gutman, (2000). Communication between individuals with dementia and their caregivers during activities of daily living. *American Journal of Alzheimer's Disease and Other Dementias* 18. 291–316.

Snowdon, D., Kemper, S., Mortimer, J., Greiner, L., Wekstein, D. & Mardesbery, W. (1996). Linguistic Ability in Early Life and Cognitive Function and Alzheimer's disease in Late Life: Findings from the Nun Study. *Journal of the American Medical Association, 275*(7), 528–33.

van Weert, J. C. M., A. M. van Dulmen, P. M. M. Spreeuwenberg, M. W. Ribbe & J. M. Bensing. (2005). Effects of snoezelen, intergrated in 24 h dementia care, on nurse–patient communication during morning care. *Patient Education and Counseling* 58(3). 312–26.

White, D. L. L. Newton-Curtas & K. S. Lyons. (2008). Development and initial testing of a measure of person-directed care. *Gerontologist* 18(1). 114–23.

Williams, K. (2001). *Improving Nursing Home Communication.* Lawrence, KS: University of Kansas dissertation. Dissertation Abstracts International 62 (UMI No. 3018543).

—, (2005). *Communication Style and Nursing Home Culture: Facility, Staff, & Resident Predictors of Elderspeak.* Paper presented at the 58th Annual Scientific Meeting of the Gerontological Society of America, Orlando, Florida, November, 18–22, 2005.

—, (2006). Improving outcomes of nursing home interactions. *Research in Nursing and Health* 29. 121–33.

Williams, K., & Herman, R. (In press). Linking resident behavior to dementia care communication: Effects of emotional tone. *Behavior Therapy.*

Williams, K. R. Herman, B. Gajewski & K. Wilson. (2009). Elderspeak communication: Impact on dementia care. *American Journal of Alzheimer's Disease and Other Dementias* 24. 11–20.

Williams, K., T. Ilten & H. Bower. (2005). Meeting communication needs: Topics of talk in the nursing home. *Journal of Psychosocial Nursing and Mental Health Services* (43). 38–45.

Williams, K., S. Kemper & M. L. Hummert. (2003). Improving nursing home communication: An intervention to reduce elderspeak. *The Gerontologist* 43(2). 242–7.

Williams, K.. & C. A. B. Warren. (2009). Communication in assisted living. *Journal of Aging Studies* 23(1). 24–36.

Chapter 2

Dementia Care Communication in Residential Facilities: Intersections of Training and Research

Boyd H. Davis and Mary K. Smith

Introduction

This paper highlights some of the ways in which corpus-based linguistic research on pragmatics and discourse of persons with dementia can be translated into communications interventions, emphasizing what the speaker with dementia retains and how that speaker can be sustained (Davis 2005). Such interventions can then be used to develop evidence-based training sequences and a curriculum for formal and informal caregivers, particularly unlicensed assistive personnel or certified nursing assistants. As we develop training, we find new research questions to bring to our corpus of talk by and with persons who have dementia of the Alzheimer's type (DAT); our efforts to better understand the nature of disordered talk elicited by the application of training and interventions lead us, in turn, to deeper research. Our examples will be drawn from our ongoing collection and study of language and dementia in assisted living residential facilities, a setting which Hyde et al. (2007) and Buckwalter et al. (2009) call "highly unstable environments" for researchers because of constant staff turnover, among other features.

After introducing the Carolinas Conversations Collection, our resource corpus, we discuss four specific examples of interactions between training and research: (i) seeing pauses as pragmatic compensation by the impaired speaker which has an impact on caregiver conversation management, (ii) co-constructing or "quilting" narrative in caregiver conversation with impaired speakers, (iii) caregivers' substituting indirect questions for wh-questions, and (iv) developing a caregiver training curriculum incorporating these techniques. We end with a series of recommendations for developing research-based interventions.

Background

Assisted living sites are designed to serve as communities for older adults wanting to age in a place where they can receive assistance as needed with activities of daily living, such as dressing, eating and/or social engagement. The sites may or may not incorporate dedicated special care dementia units in parallel or semi-detached facilities. Many—an unknown number—of assisted living residents have some degree of dementia. Indeed, Smith et al. (2008) estimate that perhaps 68% of assisted living residents have dementia.

Assisted living is a relatively new phenomenon. Hyde et al. (2007: 51) report that, "as an industry" in the United States, assisted living is only about 20 years old, and that assisted living and other types of long-term care residences differ from nursing homes in a number of ways, including a lack of common standards for staffing and for staff training. The Eldercare Locator of the U.S. Department of Health and Human Services explains that:

> Assisted living facilities may be part of a retirement community, nursing home, senior housing complex, or may stand-alone. Licensing requirements for assisted living facilities vary by state and can be known by as many as 26 different names including: residential care, board and care, congregate care, and personal care. (Eldercare Locator 2010)

As Kang et al. (2010: 19) note, "Ironically, many of the same features that make AL [assisted living] attractive to older adults, including increased privacy, choice, and the absence of federally determined care policies that permit a more homelike and less 'institutional' climate, have raised important questions about the adequacy of assisted living care for those with cognitive impairment and/or dementia diagnoses."

We have found, over the last 12 years of working with assisted living communities in North Carolina, that assisted living staff are increasingly interested in learning more about dementia, about dementia care, and about dementia care communication; administrators and families have generously allowed us to record conversations with residents, though only occasionally with staff, since administrators are concerned about disapproval by families and relocation of residents should recordings of staff-resident interactions seem negative. The conversations with residents have been preserved as one cohort within the corpus called the Carolinas Conversations Collection. When we refer to residents, it is by the alias they have within that corpus.

The Carolinas Conversations Collection: A Resource Corpus

As speakers age, their language production changes. Digital oral corpora allow researchers access to that production, including cultural, social, and interpersonal pragmatic phenomena (Pope and Davis 2010), and the intersection of sociophonetic and pragmatic features (Davis and Maclagan 2009), as well as lexicon, morphology, and syntax (Mahlberg 2005). We have based our interventions on research with materials now deposited in the password-protected Carolinas Conversations Collection hosted by the Medical Library of the Medical University of South Carolina, under the sponsorship of the National Libraries of Medicine and the National Institutes of Health.[1]

The Collection should be available to researchers in 2011. It includes transcribed audio and video interviews with two cohorts of people who are 60 years and older:

- 72+ people, 60 years and older, with DAT (longitudinal, 1998 to present), talking with researchers or students (roughly 400 conversational interviews; the majority of the speakers have moderate and late-moderate dementia);
- 72+ people, 60 years and older, with other chronic conditions (2008 to present), talking with health care graduate students and

again with community partners (roughly 150 conversational interviews; speakers have a range of medical conditions, including cancer, diabetes, and heart diseases).

There are to date about 400 conversational interviews in the Carolinas Conversations Collection with persons who have DAT. They include conversations with researchers and also with undergraduate students visiting one of four assisted living sites as part of an introductory course (Hancock et al. 2008): two are special-care assisted living facilities for people with dementia, one is an assisted living facility, and the last is an assisted living facility with an attached memory-care unit. The students receive introductory information about dementia communication and are trained in the use of several conversation-sustaining techniques discussed further in Extract (2). They are then asked to record at least one interaction, which will become part of the Carolinas Conversations Collection. Researchers can examine how persons with DAT interact in intergenerational conversations that have nothing to do with tasks in daily living, and may analyze interaction across gender, age, and ethnicity during a particular semester or year.

Changes in Pauses over Time

Our first example of interventions drawn from the study of conversational interviews in the Carolinas Conversations Collection is keyed to the intersection of pragmatic and sociophonetic features used for narrative-in-conversation (Norrick 2000, 2005). The discourse of persons with DAT changes as the disease progresses. In mild DAT, the person begins to have problems with word-finding and may ask repetitive questions; in moderate DAT, the person repeats stories, statements, favorite words, and activities and may make up stories to account for memory gaps or become accusatory; and in severe DAT, the person is difficult to understand or follow (ADEAR 2009). However, our emphasis is on retention rather than on deficit, and on what can be learned in order to help the person with DAT maintain communication with others for as long as possible (Davis 2005).

Our data from interactions by people with DAT show changes in function for the kinds of pauses in a story, and in its subsequent retelling. The use of pauses moves from signaling difficulty in finding words, typical of early and early/moderate DAT, to signaling problems with finding key components in the thread of the story, typical of late/moderate and late DAT (Davis and Maclagan 2009). In addition to their use in planning discourse, we find that pauses, fillers, and placeholders can also act as signals of 'compensation at work' (Ripich et al. 2000). We have conducted several studies (Davis and Maclagan 2010 in press; Maclagan and Davis 2010) to examine when and how the production of pauses is keyed to functions within a conversation, or to a location in the interaction, or to functions in the narrative, particularly in replacing or augmenting a defective narrative component.

In Extract (1) below, Glory Mason is recounting a story about courtship in rural areas in the early twentieth century; in Extract (2) she is recalling actions taken by members of her tiny country church concerning foot-washing, a practice followed in a number of Christian denominations to demonstrate humility and love.

Extract (2) seems to us to be an account rather than a narrative, though it includes several "small stories" in the sense used by Bamberg and Georgakopoulou (2008: 381) of "underrepresented narrative activities" that largely go unnoticed, though they are the tip of something larger, longer, and perhaps richer. In Extract (2) the phrase "my grandparents—they belonged to that church" indexes a wealth of cultural memory: Glory Mason tells us that she and her family attended there on occasion, but holding regular membership was a commitment on the part of her grandparents to the denomination, the congregation, and their beliefs and practices. This "small story" leads into her recollection of what may have been an annual or traditional ceremony involving the full congregation, whose "dinner on the ground" would have been shareable baskets of good food, held on the church lawn or side fields, probably including children's games and later, choral singing.

In these examples, the very brief pauses suggest what would be written as regular punctuation (i.e., commas and full stops) as well as marking Glory Mason's word-finding, while the slightly longer pauses of less than two seconds signal new components in both the narrative and the account. Long pauses indicate afterthought, coda (a final, closing clause in a narrative), or, as in Extract (2), a search for a missing component.[2]

(1)

- -- mother told me I had to leave my date and go milk the cows [Orientation] (laughter) come back
- -- then I wanted to eat my breakfast [Complicating action]
- -- so I asked him to come and eat [Resolution]
- -- that's the way we done it [Evaluation]
- --- boyfriend was named Burt

(2)

- - and they washed each other's feet they didn't really wash them
- - they'd pick up water in their hands and
- - they'd pour it on the feet and
- - uh
- - we attended down there some too
- - - my grandparents
- - they belonged to that church
- - - - it seemed like they did have
- - I about forgot how it was
- - they might did have a
- - foot washing in the summer time and have a
- - dinner out on the ground

In both the narrative and the account, Glory Mason is using pauses to hold the floor and keep the hearer's attention while she gets the next component ready. She is using pauses as placeholders: the hearer expects a new word to follow the very brief pauses, a new narrative component to follow the two-second pauses, and some sort of reflective commentary or parenthetical additional information after the longer pauses. Her pause patternings help her compensate for her slowed production speed and mark where the listener should wait.

The more we learn about compensatory techniques used by speakers with DAT, the more interventions we can devise for training purposes. Investigating social-interactional functions for discourse features can contribute to current discussions of the social construction of dementia and dementia care policies. Learning easy interventions involving language can help professional and family caregivers and care providers to avoid what Sabat (2006) calls the "malignant social positioning" that limits the DAT speaker to being seen merely as a patient. Accordingly, interventions that we present in our training sequences include training in wait-time: three seconds for a word-finding pause, and up to nine seconds for a story component pause, before offering the word or a suggested story component.

Quilting a Story

Paraphrase, repetition, and echo are all recommended for communication with older persons who suffer from confusion or dementia (Dijkstra et al. 2002; Bourgeois 2002). Our ongoing analysis of paraphrase, repetition and phatic communication in Alzheimer's discourse identifies their intersection with formulaic phrases (Wray 2008), particularly those which occur in efforts to produce a story. Accordingly, we developed "quilting" (Moore and Davis 2002) as a co-construction technique which can be taught quickly to caregivers and inserted into daily care routines, but which has impact beyond the surface.

Quilting involves caregivers co-constructing personal stories over several encounters with the impaired person. This co-construction supports retention of multiple facets of identity for the impaired person and, at least anecdotally, reduces agitation. Quilting allows staff to expand daily care routines and develop list-making and facilitated poetry activities. Such activities tap earlier skills in categorization and tabulation, and activate implicit memory. In the following two conversations with Robbie Walters, we see the researcher eliciting details on one occasion, shown in Extract (3), and presenting a key detail about Nitro, a town in West Virginia, on the next occasion, two weeks later, shown in Extract (4):

(3)

B:	Who's in the pictures?
ROBBIE:	Those are just up there on that wall from this building. I'm not -- I don't know them
B:	You don't know those people?
ROBBIE:	They're of other people
B:	Uh-huh.
ROBBIE:	I did
B:	Oh, OK

ROBBIE: have sisters
- - There's Muffin, my little poodle

B: Oh, Muffin, the poodle. What color poodle was she?

ROBBIE: White
- - and
- - we went on the hill up there from Nitro a good bit

B: A dog is such a comfort

ROBBIE: You sure do miss them

In Extract (3), the researcher brings up Nitro, which elicits a great many more details from Walters, details which will be used to construct even more narratives, particularly about his wartime service, over the following several months.

(4)

B: The last time we were here you were talking about going up on the hill above Nitro and looking out over the valley

ROBBIE: Yeah, well I used to do that in the younger years, earlier
- - Yeah
- - But yes
- I used to look
- overlook the Monsanto and the chemical companies there that was in the valley
- yeah

B: Did you work there?

ROBBIE: No
- not at Monsanto but at Viscose
- I was right next to it.

B: Oh
- Ok

ROBBIE: but I
- - I did work at the Viscose plant for a short period of time and then I went into the military

Over the next 18 months, researchers visiting Robbie Walters were able to co-construct with him a more expanded story about his wartime experiences in World War II. If we assume the life span perspective on reminiscence put forth by Baltes (1987), as suggested in Webster et al. (2010: 532), we see that quilting as an activity supports Baltes' proposition that reminiscence development extends across the life span and can support flashes of lucidity and recall.

Further study of the construction and co-construction of reminiscence narratives, accounts, and small stories can be supported by the conversational interviews in the Carolinas Conversations Collection, and will allow further examination of what Webster et al. (2010: 537) call moderators—that is, "variables that can potentially influence reminiscence occurrence, process, and outcome," and which include gender, age, and ethnicity. For example, the initial analysis by Davis and Nold (2004) of conversations with Robbie Walters found that he apparently retained gender-based expectations about who could ask questions and understand answers keyed to wartime military experiences. When talking to Davis, an American woman with only a few personal memories of childhood in World War II, Walters presented general statements about his war service and his work in Europe, whereas when talking to Nold—a European man who by life experience as a child in wartime and postwar Germany could ask specific questions—Walters proffered many details, sometimes without having been prompted or asked for them.

Research Leading to Intervention: Using Indirect Questions

Neurological research suggests that cognitive processing costs are less when the speaker can recognize a topic, rather than retrieve an answer to a question (Kempler 2005). Our ongoing analysis of question-answer interactions and their pragmatic impact has led to additional research on the interaction of discourse markers with pauses and filled pauses, as well as to our beginning to develop training that enables caregivers to change their question-asking habits and to move from an over-dependence on the wh-question to other ways of soliciting information or initiating conversation.

Whether the interruption by a wh-question is a disruption of working memory or semantic memory, both disrupt the allocation of attention. Givón (1993: 191) comments that: "Questions can be used to present certain things as given, as facts. This works best of all with wh-questions, because almost everything in them except for the wh-item is presupposed." Looking at wh-questions allows researchers to "test theoretical accounts in order to gain a more detailed insight into the underlying nature of aphasia," say Salis and Edwards (2008: 376, 378), adding that who/what-questions are thought to be less demanding than which-questions.

Kempler et al. (1998: 61) claim that "patients with Alzheimer's disease can successfully process sentences with relatively complex meanings as they hear them. Therefore, these patients' sentence comprehension deficits are likely due to an inability to maintain active information in memory and not due to a purely semantic impairment." Partee (2009) notes that researchers make distinctions among syntactic, semantic, and pragmatic notions of what a question is. We suggest that any of these distinctions may contribute to the problems speakers with DAT face in storing a question in working memory, in retrieving an answer which will correspond to the demands of the syntactic form, semantic content, and pragmatic appropriateness for the question, in rematching the answer to the questions, and in producing the answer.

Ferstl et al. (2005) used a story test to identify comprehension deficits after brain damage, using yes-no questions, which allowed the comparison of responses to questions about stated versus implied information. Questions about main ideas were easier than details; questions about explicit information were easier than about implicit information. Whereas Singer (2003) outlined discourse comprehension theory and reviewed processing stages, including parallel processing models and global memory search, our own interest focuses on variation in production and sociopragmatic contexts for talk. Over the past three years, Boyd H. Davis, the first author of this paper, has been working with other colleagues to mine the same corpus for the interaction among pauses, fillers, and discourse or pragmatic markers in three contexts, the findings of which can be adapted for our present training materials.

Context (1) is an analysis of the use of pauses, fillers, and pragmatic markers in conversations on similar topics with older persons from the United States who have no cognitive impairment compared with same-gender, same-ethnicity unimpaired speakers from New Zealand (Davis and Maclagan 2010). These conversational interviews are in the Carolinas Conversations Collection and in the ONZE Miner collection. One finding to date is that in the speech of unimpaired speakers (i.e., both interviewer and narrator), regardless of national English variations, the pragmatic uses of a marker such as "So" are always accompanied by a pause. Most often the pause precedes the "So" (occasionally it follows it), and the pause is usually relatively long. The uses include the initiation of a new discourse unit or topic, the resumption of a discourse unit or topic, and a closure sequence of turns that typically includes an evaluative comment which is often a formulaic phrase.

Context (2) is an analysis of the use of pauses, fillers, and pragmatic markers in conversations with persons from the U.S. and from New Zealand (Davis and Maclagan 2011 in press) who have cognitive impairment. Again, these conversational interviews are drawn from the Carolinas Conversations Collection and the ONZE Miner collection. One finding is that placeholders, fillers, and formulaic sequences are still used appropriately and help cement interaction by providing appropriate cues to the conversational partner.

Context (3) constitutes a preliminary analysis of the interaction of pauses, fillers, and pragmatic markers with question-types, comparing the production by unimpaired and by impaired older persons who are conversing while sitting and conversing while walking (Karakostas et al. 2010; Maclagan and Davis 2010). To date, we have identified a cline of difficulty in language production by question type for both unimpaired and impaired speakers, with a stronger trend for speakers with DAT, particularly when walking. Not surprisingly, the initial finding is that the greatest difficulty is in responding to wh-questions.

This set of related studies reinforces our belief that studying the speech of people with DAT may provide insights into how cognitively impaired speakers continue trying to make meaning with their conversation partners. Such study may also provide insights into unimpaired speech, in that what is retained and manipulated may contribute not only to studies of listener expectations about speaker competencies, but also to studies of both the acquisition and the loss of particular language features. And finally, it reminds us that no question is ever innocent.

Accordingly, we support the use of dementia care communications interventions such as those outlined by Dijkstra et al. (2002: 153), namely that of "using short sentences or instructions during care routines, giving positive feedback to the resident when responding to an instruction, giving the resident sufficient time to respond to an instruction or question (five seconds), talking about the resident's life or hobbies, and avoiding unhelpful questions." We have also introduced the intervention of the indirect question (as well as the tag and the yes-no question) as preferable to wh-questions, with training and reinforcement such as the following:

INSTEAD OF . . .

– Asking direct questions starting with *Who, What, Do you, Did you,* such as:
  What do you think about . . .?
  Who is the man in this picture?
  Do you remember how many children . . .?

TRY . . .

– Rephrasing as a statement or yes-no question, such as:
  You had two sisters, I believe . . .
  You had two sisters, didn't you . . .
  So, you have two sisters.
– Introducing your "question" with a word such as *So* or *Well,* which tells the listener that you are going to summarize or ask something.

The response from caregiver trainees to this particular intervention has been interesting: offering what seems like a statement instead of a direct wh-question seems to them a new concept. However, with minimal practice, such as in role-playing situations, caregivers report that they elicit positive responses from residents and that they do so with greater ease.

Web-delivered Content in Hybrid or Blended Training

Since 2005, we have been drawing on the conversational interviews and the findings from research studying these interviews to refine an Internet-delivered curriculum for certified nursing assistants and a set of materials on culturally sensitive and culturally competent dementia care communication for nurses. The development and initial evaluation of the curriculum and materials was funded by the Alzheimer's Association.

The materials draw on audio and video conversations now housed in the Carolinas Conversations Collection, particularly for the critical writing prompts and the vignettes that accompany each of the 16 units on basic skills in caregiving in the certified nursing assistants' curriculum, and the modules for nurses, which have been specifically tailored to communication and dementia care. Vignettes include situations keyed to conversation and may include links to audio or video transcripts, such as the following conversational exchange, Extract (5) (cited in Davis and Pope 2009), that illustrates sensitive ways to handle a resident's confusion about time.

(5)

LW: They got a lot of
-- they got a lot of rosewoods on the stop.
LM: A lot of rosebuds on the stop?
LW: Yeah.
LM: Ummm.
LW: --- That's going to be awfully pretty when they open that up!
LM: Oh absolutely!
LW: Yeah.
LM: You like rosebuds too?
LW: That's my favorite!
LM: That makes you happy, doesn't it? Did you have a bunch of rose bushes when you were growing up? Did your Mama plant rose bushes?
LW: My mother had awfully pretty ones this year.
LM: She did? This year?
LW: She won't let me get in them! She's afraid I'll trim it up!

Since LW is becoming more severely affected by dementia, LM, the researcher, does not correct him; instead she remodels, substituting rosebuds for rosewoods within an indirect question asking for clarification. As the conversation continues, LM asks direct questions about whether his mother had planted roses. LW continues to contribute to the conversation, talking about his mother's roses "this year." Since LW is in his late eighties, LM offers him a chance, with an echo question, to readjust his time perspective. Since he remains in the time perspective of his mother's gardening, she again does not correct him but moves instead to a new topic.

We have been heartened by learners' response to our new materials on dementia care communication. The materials are currently delivered as the online component of classes that blend online and face-to-face interaction and are tailored to accommodate a range of fluencies in the learners. We emphasize vignettes and story lines, because they enable us to build in cultural components and illustrate cultural contexts for social interaction. Test scores by 400 students across three years, in fifteen different classes and seven different instructors, are encouraging. After implementation of the enhanced materials, nursing assistant student outcomes at certification level produced pass rates for nurse aide certification that increased to 90% on average across 15 classes; their previous pass rate had been 80%. Instructors report a greater retention in second-language learners due to accessibility of materials and ability to practice and repeat, and an advance in language skills (predominantly in reading) by an average of 2 years per student as demonstrated in standardized pre- and post-testing using the Test of Adult Basic Education (Davis et al. 2008; Davis and Smith 2009). An online survey[3] indicated the nursing assistant students viewed the enhanced materials positively.

We have found that students improve in writing fluency as well as in speaking proficiency. We used CPIDR (Computerized Propositional Idea Density Rater), a tool based on artificial intelligence (see Covington 2009) to measure propositional density (Brown et al. 2008) in extemporaneous written recounts of goals (at the beginning of the training course) and clinical experiences (at the end of the course). Density increased, though it was not significant. The change in the kinds of words used for extemporaneous recounts of experience, however, were that second-language as well as first-language nurse aide students increased their use of both academic and technical/medical vocabulary, as analyzed by an online Vocabulary Profiler (Cobb 2009). Using the new vocabulary in their writing suggests that the students would have an increased understanding of directions and information about healthcare and patient safety given by their supervisors.

Recommendations for Practitioners

When we analyzed caregiver talk with persons suffering from DAT, using the seven characteristics of therapeutic language originally identified by Ferrara (1994), we observed that speaker parity soon became lost (Davis and Pope 2009). With speakers who have DAT, parity is suspended—the caregiver has symbolic capital, and the other has not. Until other factors, including cultural expectations, are introduced, unmarked or casual acts in ordinary conversation start with both parties assumed to have parity. With a therapist, the patient agrees to enter an unequal relationship with assigned roles for who will talk and who will listen, and thus who will regulate and terminate interaction. This is clearly not the case with institutional residents with DAT. As for caregiver-resident interactions, research shows that most caregiver communication is task directed, meaning that caregivers focus on the residents' daily/functional activities and physical health, as well as on their own concerns (Iwasiw and Olson 1995). Patient-initiated reminiscences, hopes, plans are often ignored (Davis and Pope 2009; Davis and Smith 2009; Hamilton 1994, 2008a, 2008b; Ramanathan 1997, 2008).

According to Allen-Burge et al. (2001: 215), "[institutional] residents who are impaired in cognition, sensory functioning, and communication are at risk for spending little to no time with other residents," which makes them even more dependent on interactions with caregivers. However, Burgio et al. (2002) note that the average time per day of social interaction via communication is a scant four minutes. Moreover, common caregiver practices include talking for, talking over, and talking across the person with dementia. Caregivers thereby provide only task-related, instrumental care, which, by leaving the door open to social neglect, is one step away from being abusive (Davis and Pope 2009).

When caregiving staff are involved in implementing hands-on activities with residents and encouraging social interaction among them, they are practicing a patient-centered care that stems from an evidence-based training. The 2007 report prepared by the Institute for the Future of Aging Services, entitled *The long-term care workforce: Can the crisis be fixed?* (IFAS 2007: 16), lists Goal 4 as: "Make Larger and Smarter Investments in the Development and Continuing Education of the Long-Term Care Workforce" (IFAS 2007: 16). This goal asks for a redesign of training that could help offset high job turnover in assisted living. Included in this goal is the objective of making training more accessible with techniques including Web-based courses. In addition to endorsing such a technique, particularly since we are using and finding Web-based materials successful for training delivery, we end our discussion with ten recommendations for the development of training materials.

Practical Implications

Ten recommendations for dementia communication training materials:

1. Dementia communication training should foster a person-centered caregiving that goes beyond task-oriented, minimal care.
2. Dementia care training should demonstrate how to involve communication with every activity of daily living.
3. Dementia communication techniques must be able to be demonstrated easily and taught quickly, with minimal rehearsal.
4. Dementia communication techniques must be internalized by the caregiver and seen as capable of being part of daily routines. Ideally, techniques will work the first time they are tried, and will usually get notable positive response in terms of patient mood, attitude, or compliance. If considered as interventions, measurable outcomes will be easily identified.
5. Ideally, materials and training will incorporate peer-reviewed techniques and will have measurable outcomes emphasizing patient safety and quality of life.
6. Training materials for adult learners need to be presented in multiple media to engage attention and sustain retention.
7. Given migration patterns for older people, domestics, entry-level health care workers, and nurses (de Bot and Makoni 2005), training materials need to be easy to translate, and multilingual whenever possible.
8. Materials should, whenever possible, be derived from a research program in real-world settings.
9. Materials and training in the United States must contribute to the call for new policies governing social interaction and communication for persons with dementia (Saliba and Buchanan 2008).
10. Training materials should be designed to accommodate academic course components, certification training sequences, orientation

for new hires, as well as continuing education instructional units used for recertification of staff licensures.

Notes

[1] Initial data searches of the Carolinas Conversations Collection can be conducted by the public. The search is keyed to age, gender, race, ethnicity, first language, language of interview, and health condition. To accommodate access, retrieval and analysis, the Carolinas Conversations Collection data is mounted and delivered via Carolina Miner, an offshoot of ONZE Miner, originally developed as the data management package for the project "Origins of New Zealand English" (Fromont and Hay 2006). Users whose proposals meet criteria of institutional review boards (IRBs) at home institutions and at the Medical University of South Carolina may access the password-protected, time-aligned transcripts of audio and video recordings for download and analysis using their own preferred tools. They may also analyze them online via links in the Carolina Miner database, links to a suite of tools for acoustic analysis, lexicon, or syntax.

[2] We arranged the transcribed speech in all extracts as stanzas (Johnstone 2007) keyed to the speaker's patterns in pausing, using the following symbols:

- indicates a brief pause of less than 1 second;
-- indicates a pause of less than 2 seconds;
--- indicates a long pause of more than 2 seconds.

[3] Just under 30% (n = 68) of the students responded to the voluntary survey: 70.6% reported using the content and techniques of the communications model during their clinical experience, another 19.1% reported that they had "maybe" done so, and 94% reported that the dementia communications module had contributed to their delivering safer and more responsive patient care.

References

ADEAR (Alzheimer's Disease Education & Referral Center). (2009). *Understanding Stages and Symptoms of Alzheimer's Disease.* www.nia.nih.gov/Alzheimers/Publications/stages.htm (last accessed 10 September 2010).

Allen-Burge, R., L. Burgio, M. Bourgeois, R. Sims & J. Nunnikhoven. (2001). Increasing communication among nursing home residents. *Journal of Clinical Geropsychology* 7. 213–30.

Baltes, P. (1987). Theoretical propositions of life-span developmental psychology: On the dynamics between growth and decline. *Developmental Psychology* 23. 611–26.

Bamberg, M. & A. Georgakopoulou. (2008). Small stories as a new perspective in narrative and identity analysis. *Text & Talk* 28. 377–96.

Bourgeois, M. (2002). 'Where is my wife and when am I going home?': The challenge of communicating with persons with dementia. *Alzheimer's Care Quarterly* 3. 132–44.

Brown, C., T. Snodgrass, S. Kemper, R. Herman & M. Covington. (2008). Automatic measurement of propositional idea density from part-of-speech tagging. *Behavioral Research Methods* 40. 540–5.

Buckwalter, K., M. Grey, B. Bowers, A. M. McCarthy, D. Gross, M. Funk & C. Beck. (2009). Intervention research in highly unstable environments. *Research in Nursing & Health* 32). 110–21.

Burgio, L. D., A. Stevens, K. L. Burgio, D. L. Roth, P. Paul & J. Gerstle. (2002). Teaching and maintaining behavior management skills in the nursing home. *The Gerontologist* 42. 487–96.

Cobb, T. (2009). Web Vocabprofile, adapted from A. Heatley and P. Nation's Range. Accessed 10 December 2009 at www.lextutor.ca/vp/

Covington, M. A. (2009). *Idea Density: A Potentially Useful Characteristic of Retrieved Documents.* www.ai.uga.edu/caspr/Covington-2009-Idea-Density-paper-SEC09–060.pdf (last accessed February 2010).

Davis, B. (ed.). (2005). *Alzheimer Talk, Text and Context: Enhancing Communication.* New York: Palgrave.

Davis, B. & M. Maclagan. (2009). Examining pauses in Alzheimer's discourse. *American Journal of Alzheimer's Disease and Other Dementias* 24. 141–54.

—(2010). Pauses, fillers, placeholders and formulaicity in Alzheimer's discourse: Gluing relationships as impairment increases. In N. Amiridze, B. Davis & M. Maclagan (eds), *Fillers, Pauses, and Placeholders,* 189–215. Amsterdam: John Benjamins.

—(2011 in press). Stylistic usage of pragmatic markers and habituated pauses: Performative functions retained by older speakers. In M. Macaulay and P. Blitvich (eds), *Pragmatics and Contexts.* Toronto: Antares.

Davis, B. & G. Nold. (2004). Twice-told tales: War stories and Alzheimer's speakers. *Language and Aging Symposium,* International Conference in Language & Social Psychology, June 2004, Pennsylvania State University.

Davis, B. & C. Pope. (2009). Institutionalized ghosting: Policy contexts and language use in erasing the person with Alzheimer's. *Language Policy* 9. 29–44.

Davis, B, L. Russell-Pinson & M. Smith. (2008). Collaboration in ESP: Towards a multilingual, multicultural nursing assistant workforce. *ESP Across Cultures* (5). 7–22.

Davis, B. & M. Smith. (2009). Infusing cultural competence training into the curriculum: Describing the development of culturally sensitive training on dementia communication. *Kaohsiung Journal of Medical Sciences* (25). 503–9.

de Bot, K. & S. Makoni. (2005). *Language and Aging in Multilingual Settings.* Clevedon, U.K.: Multilingual Matters.

Dijkstra, K., M. Bourgeois, L. Burgio, R. Allen. (2002). Effects of a communication intervention on the discourse of nursing home residents with nursing assistants. *Journal of Medical Speech-Language Pathology* (10). 143–58.

Eldercare Locator. (2010). *Assisted Living,* fact sheets. www.eldercare.gov/Eldercare.NET/Public/Resources/fact_sheets/assisted_living.aspx (last accessed 10 September 2010).

Ferrara. K. (1994). *Therapeutic Ways With Words.* Oxford: Oxford University Press.

Ferstl, E., K. Walther, T. Guthke & D. von Cramon. (2005). Assessment of story comprehension deficits after brain damage. *Journal of Clinical and Experimental Neuropsychology* (27). 367–84.

Fromont, R. & J. Hay. (2006) *ONZEMiner.* For ONZE (Origins of New Zealand English) Project, in the Linguistics Department of the University of Canterbury, Christchurch, New Zealand. Accessed June 30, 2008, www.ling.canterbury.ac.nz/jen/onzeminer/

Givón, T. (1993). *English grammar: A function-based introduction,* volume II. Philadelphia: John Benjamins.

Hamilton, H. (1994). *Conversations With an Alzheimer's Patient: An interactional sociolinguistic study.* Cambridge: Cambridge University Press.

—(2008a). Language and dementia: Sociolinguistic aspects. *Annual Review of Applied Linguistics* 28. 91–110.

—(2008b). Narrative as snapshot: Glimpses of the past in Alzheimer talk. *Narrative Inquiry* 18. 53–82.

Hancock, C., D. Shenk & B. Davis. (2008). Integrating gerontology service-learning students as members of a research team. In M. Moore & P. Lan Lim (eds), *Service Learning in Higher Education: Paradigms and Challenges,* 171–84. University of Indianapolis Press

Hyde, J., R. Perez & B. Forester. (2007). Dementia and assisted living. *Gerontologist* 47. 51–67.

IFAS (Institute for the Future of Aging Services). (2007). *The Long-term Care Workforce: Can the Crisis be Fixed? Problems, Causes and Options.* www.aahsa.org/uploadedFiles/IFAS/Publications_amp;_Products/LTCCommission Report2007.pdf (last accessed 10 September 2010).

Iwasiw, C. & J. Olson. (1995). Content analysis of nonprofessional caregiver-patient interactions in long-term care facilities. *Clinical Nursing Research* 4. 411–24.

Johnstone, B. (2007). *Discourse Analysis,* 2nd edn Malden, MA: Blackwell.

Kang H., M. Smith, K. Buckwalter, V. Ellingrod & S. Schultz. (2010). Anxiety, depression, and cognitive impairment in dementia-specific and traditional assisted living. *Journal of Gerontological Nursing* (36). 19–30.

Karakostas, T., B. Davis, M. Maclagan & S. Hsiang. (2010). Walking and conversing: Gait and speech adaptations to perturbing direct questions in dementia. *Parkinsonism and Related Disorders* 16(1). S11–S86, S49.

Kempler, D. (2005). *Neurocognitive Disorders in Aging.* Thousand Oaks, CA: Sage Publishers.

Kempler, D., A. Almor & M. MacDonald. (1998). Teasing apart the contribution of memory and language impairments in Alzheimer's disease. *American Journal of Speech-Language Pathology* 7. 61–7.

Maclagan, M. & B. Davis. (2010). Conversing while sitting: The impact of different question types on conversation. *Poster Presentation.* Auckland, NZ: New Zealand Speech Therapy Association.

Mahlberg, M. (2005). *English General Nouns: A Corpus Theoretical Approach.* Amsterdam: John Benjamins.

Moore, L. & B. Davis. (2002). Quilting narrative: Using repetition techniques to help elderly communicators. *Geriatric Nursing* 23. 262–6.

Norrick, N. (2000). *Conversational Narrative: Storytelling in Everyday Talk.* Amsterdam: John Benjamins.

—(2005). Interactional remembering in conversational narrative. *Journal of Pragmatics* 37. 1819–44.

Partee, B. (2009). *Lecture 11 (Week 12): Semantics and Pragmatics of Questions* (Formal Semantics, MGU, May 22, 2009). http://people.umass.edu/partee/MGU_2009/materials/MGU0911.pdf *(last accessed 10 September 2010).*

Pope, C. & B. Davis. (2010 in press.) Finding a balance: The Carolinas Conversations Collection. *Corpus Linguistics and Linguistic Theory.*

Ramanathan, V. (1997). *Alzheimer Discourse: Some Sociolinguistic Dimensions.* Mahwah, NJ: Lawrence Erlbaum.

—(2008). Applied linguistics redux: A Derridean exploration of Alzheimer life histories. *Applied Linguistics* 29. 1–23.

Ripich, D., B. Carpenter & E. Ziol. (2000). Conversational cohesion patterns in men and women with Alzheimer's disease: A longitudinal study. *Brain and Language* 35. 49–64.

Sabat, S. (2006). Mind, meaning and personhood in dementia: the effects of positioning. In J. Hughes, S. Louw, & S. Sabat (eds), *Dementia: Mind, Meaning and the Person,* 287–301. Oxford: Oxford University Press.

Saliba, D. & J. Buchanan. (2008). *Development and Validation of a Revised Nursing Home Assessment Tool: MDS 3.0.* Baltimore: Rand. Accessed 14 December 2008 at *www.cms.hhs.gov/nursinghomequalityinits/25_nhqimds30.asp*

Salis, C. & S. Edwards. (2008). Comprehension of wh-questions and declarative sentences in agrammatic aphasia: The set partition hypothesis. *Journal of Neurolinguistics* 21. 375–99.

Singer, M. (2003). Processes of question answering. In G. Rickheit, T. Herrmann & W. Deutsch (eds), *Psycholinguistik/Psycholinguistics,* 422–31. Berlin: Walter de Gruyter.

Smith, M., K. C. Buckwalter, H. Kang, V. Ellingrod & S. K. Schultz. (2008). Dementia care in assisted living: Needs and challenges. *Issues in Mental Health Nursing* 29. 817–38.

Webster, J., E. Bohlmeijer & G. Westerhof. (2010). Mapping the future of reminiscence: A conceptual guide for research and practice. *Research on Aging* 32. 537–64.

Wray, A. (2008). *Formulaic Language: Pushing the Boundaries.* Oxford: Oxford University Press.

Chapter 3

Creating a Positive Communication Environment in Long-Term Care

Rosemary Lubinski

Introduction

We are aging globally. In 2006, there were 500 million people worldwide aged 65 years and above, and this figure will double by 2030 (Senior Journal 2009). Each of these older persons will at some point face the question of whether to live independently in the community or relocate to a more supportive environment that meets their changing physical, mental, social, and financial needs. Most older persons reside in the community; however, with aging and an increase in disability, the need for relocation to some type of long-term care facility increases. According to conservative estimates, 5% of those over 65 years of age reside in skilled nursing facilities, and this increases to 21% for those aged 85 and older (Stone 2000). In the United States at least 1.4 million people, most of them older, reside in about 18,000 skilled nursing facilities (Senior Journal 2009).

Today, there are a number of living options beyond the family home that provide an array of services to meet increasing needs. Living facilities provide room, board, and supervision, and some degree of socialization, housekeeping, personal care, medical care, and rehabilitation. Some older persons may need the minimal care provided in settings such as group homes and assisted living facilities that encourage autonomy and independence. Others may benefit from full-time care in skilled nursing facilities that tend to be more restrictive and institutional. A growing number of residential campuses offer a continuum of care, and older residents can move from one level of care to another as their needs change.

Regardless of the type of long-term care setting in which older persons reside, communication is critical to their well-being. Older residents who can communicate effectively maximize their independence, maintain their connection with family and others, receive quality care, and enhance their sense of self-worth and dignity. In addition, when residents can communicate successfully, professional caregivers can naturally incorporate affective care and perform their tasks more efficiently and effectively. Successful communication also encourages family members to visit and to engage older residents in conversations that are meaningful to both parties.

Professionals interested in creating a positive communication environment for older persons in long-term care settings need a model to guide their assessment and intervention practices. This paper outlines a tripartite model that can be used as a foundation for creating a positive communication environment in such settings. It is based on three components: (i) communication skills, (ii) communication effectiveness, and (iii) communication opportunities. As will be shown, the model can be used as a template for assessment and intervention in long-term care settings. The critical role of committed and trained communication partners is emphasized as well as the necessity for modifying the physical and social environment in long-term care facilities.

Skill, Effectiveness, and Opportunity Model

A comprehensive model provides a clinically useful framework for understanding the communication of older persons in long-term care settings. The model should focus on both older residents and their family or professional caregiver communication partners. It should also consider the physical and social context in which communication occurs and have flexibility to describe communication in a variety of types of long-term care settings. Finally, the model should document the effects of intervention. The model proposed in this paper begins with understanding the communication skills of the older resident, recognizes the role of communication partners and assistive technology in fostering communication effectiveness, and appreciates the influence of the physical and social context on creating or hindering communication opportunities (Lubinski 2008).

Communication Skill

Communication skill is defined as the ability to receive, interpret, and send messages through a variety of modalities including speaking, reading, understanding, writing, and gesturing. Communication skills also include the underlying cognitive, social, and emotional skills that support interaction. Communication skills necessitate some degree of adequacy in visual and/or auditory abilities. The ability to communicate successfully requires that older persons understand what they see or hear and can formulate at least minimally understandable responses through speech, writing, drawing, other nonverbal means, or some combination of these modalities.

Communication skills change with normal aging and are complicated with the onset of a variety of disorders. For example, word retrieval ability may decrease especially over the age of 70 as does comprehension of complex syntax (Worrall and Hickson 2003). Communication discourse may show some changes including less efficiency and increased off-topic verbosity, more ambiguity, and less cohesion (Garcia and Orange 1996). Speech and vocal changes tend to be distinctive but have minimal impact on intelligibility (Worrall and Hickson 2003: 97). Although the communication changes with normal aging are relatively subtle, older persons' communication may be perceived negatively and responded to in a patronizing way (Garcia and Orange 1996). For an in-depth discussion of elderspeak, see Williams (this volume).

The onset of pathologies associated with stroke, traumatic injury, dementia, laryngectomy, and progressive neurological disorders (e.g., Parkinson's disease) has an important impact on the communication skills of older residents. Each of these will affect language and speech skills to some extent. Unfortunately, there are few recent epidemiological studies of communication disorders in long-term care facilities. In a national review of nursing home resident characteristics in the United States, Krauss and Altman (1996) found that at least 60% of residents had difficulty with expression and comprehension.

Worrall et al. (1993) in a study of 535 residents in an A
nursing home found that 43% of the residents failed an aph
58% a pragmatic test, 83% a mental test, 84% a hearing test, a
of the residents failed at least one of the communication screening tests. Further, it can be inferred through review of the common diagnoses of skilled nursing home residents that communication impairments are common, especially those related to hearing loss, stroke, dementia, and progressive neurological disorders.

Adequate vision and hearing underlie the reception of information. Blindness affects about 1% of those over age 40, and another 2% have low vision (Congdon et al. 2004). The prevalence of age-related eye diseases (ARED) increases with age. For example, cataracts, the most common ARED among older persons, affects 20% of those at age 65 but 68% of those over 80 years (National Eye Institute 2010). Other AREDs include glaucoma, macular degeneration, and diabetic retinopathy. Tielsch et al. (1995) in a vision prevalence study of nursing home patients found that the rate of blindness was 13 to 15 times higher than for community-based peers and that blindness increased with age. Older persons with stroke or head injury are at higher risk of vision impairment (Vision Help 2010). Vision impairment affects all activities of daily living as well as cognition, emotional status, and socialization.

The American Speech-Language-Hearing Association (ASHA 2004) reports that the prevalence of hearing loss increases from one in three for those aged 65–74 to one in two for those over age 85. The prevalence of hearing loss also increases among older nursing home residents (Better Hearing Institute 2009) with the results of one study indicating that as many as 77% of older residents had at least a mild hearing loss (Garahan et al. 1992). Hearing loss among those with dementia is also prevalent. Uhlmann et al. (1989) found that the prevalence of a mild hearing loss was significantly higher for those with dementia than matched controls and that hearing loss was correlated with severity of cognitive impairment. Gold et al. (1996) screened the hearing of 52 older persons and found that 49 of the 52 had a significant hearing loss.

Hearing loss has a detrimental effect on receiving information related to care and socialization and may result in confusion, depression, and withdrawal. Cassie and Rockwell (1994) found that nursing home residents with hearing loss were not able to effectively manage the conversational breakdowns they had with staff members. The Better Hearing Institute (2009) also states that fewer than half of those with significant hearing losses are identified by staff in nursing homes. Hearing loss may not only be underidentified in these settings but may contribute to older residents being misclassified as having depression, dementia, or confusion. For an excellent discussion of hearing loss and compromised cognitive skills see Kricos (2006).

Dual sensory impairment, or combined vision and hearing loss, is common among older persons in general. According to Lighthouse International (2006), at least 21% of older persons in the community have dual losses that result in greater functional disability, dissatisfaction with social interaction, greater risk of falls, more difficulties with physical functioning, and greater use of health care support. Berry et al. (2004) maintain that this "double trouble" affects communication, socialization, and independent living. Bagley (1995) states that many with dual losses acquire them late in life; the losses were "dismissed" as a part of normal aging and were not recognized as remediable.

There is an unequivocal negative impact on quality of life in a nursing home when older residents have hearing, vision, or communication problems. In a study of over 18,000 nursing homes in the United States, Resnick et al. (1997) found that hearing loss, vision impairment, and communication difficulties were all associated with less social engagement and time spent in activities.

Communication skills are also influenced by the emotional and cognitive characteristics of older residents. The prevalence of depression among nursing home residents in the United States ranges from about 20% (Jones et al. 2005) to one in three (Wagenaar et al. 2003) to 50% (AHCA 2010). A nursing home prevalence study in the Netherlands indicates that 8.1% of residents had major depression, 14.1% had minor depression, and another 24% had subclinical depression. Among the risk indicators for major depression are stroke, visual impairment, loneliness, and lack of social support, all factors associated with communication skills and opportunities

(Jongenelis et al. 2004). Similarly, depression is often an unrecognized and undertreated diagnosis (Wagenaar et al. 2003).

Dementia is one of the most common diagnoses among nursing home residents. Data collected by the Centers for Medicare and Medicaid indicate that about 47% of residents have dementia. Other studies have reported higher rates: 62% (Matthews and Deming 2002) and 67% (Rovner et al. 1990). Dementia will affect communication skills and opportunities as it progresses. In the early stage, communication is characterized by subtle changes in comprehension and expression, but as it progresses to mid-stage, communication becomes significantly compromised, particularly in conversations. In late-stage dementia, communication is severely impaired in all modalities. Of particular interest is the effect of dementia on the ability to hold a conversation. Orange and Purves (1996) state that discourse becomes more egocentric, wordy but empty, and characterized by poor discourse maintenance and relevancy. Conversational partners have difficulty repairing conversational breakdowns.

Communication Effectiveness

Communication effectiveness is characterized by the ability to receive, interpret, and send messages successfully despite message imperfection. Some older persons will not make significant improvements in their communication skills even when there is speech-language therapy provided. In some cases, older persons will have such severe communication problems—exacerbated by numerous other physical, cognitive, and emotional morbidities—that rehabilitation does not result in optimum improvement. For others, there may be insufficient access to and funding for therapy. Regardless of the reason for limited progress, older residents still need to communicate their needs and understand what is said to them. Thus, they need communication partners who themselves have skills that facilitate communication. Some residents with compromised communication skills might also benefit from the use of personal or environmental assistive communication devices.

The primary communication partners of older residents in long-term care facilities are staff members, particularly those who provide personal care on a one-to-one basis. In addition, family members have important social roles in communicating effectively with residents and staff caregivers. Both family members and caregivers are frequently challenged by the resident's communication impairments and the effects of an impoverished communication environment. A comprehensive approach to meeting the needs of these residents must incorporate professional caregivers and families.

Communication Opportunities

Communication opportunity is defined as the physical, psychosocial, linguistic, and cultural accessibility to communication partners of choice and to activities that generate meaningful conversations and interactions. Older persons may possess adequate communication skills and even have partners who can facilitate interaction, but they still need communication opportunities where they might interact and demonstrate their competency to the highest degree possible. The physical and social milieu in long-term care settings is more than a passive background but serves as an active contributor to and influence on the communication that occurs there. The communication environment in many long-term care facilities may be considered communication impaired or impoverished (Grainger 2004; Lubinski 2008).

A communication impaired environment is characterized by physical and social barriers to communicative interaction for older adults and their communication partners. Such environments share the following features (Lubinski 2008: 329):

(a) a lack of sensitivity to the value of communication as a therapeutic agent,
(b) the perception that communication is a by-product rather than a focus of care,
(c) stated or unstated rules that limit communicative interaction,
(d) a lack of communication partners of choice,
(e) limited physical access to activities and partners that engender interaction,
(f) few reasons to talk that emanate from meaningful activities and interaction,

(g) lack of communicative privacy,
(h) lack of personal or environmental sensory aids or cognitive enrichment to meet the needs of older persons,
(i) inadequate or insufficient intervention to improve impaired receptive and expressive communication skills, and
(j) little or no training and support for communication partners.

Numerous studies have delineated the communication impoverishment in long-term care facilities. A few examples are discussed here. In a study of resident perceptions of communication in a nursing home, Lubinski, Morrison, and Rigrodsky (1981) found that, despite the perceived lack of meaningful communication opportunities, residents still wanted to talk. The authors stated, "Communication occurs, but they [i.e., the residents] perceive that others do more talking than themselves. When they do talk, it centers on a narrow range of topics and occurs in public places. Residents want to talk, enjoy it, and generally feel that their status would be enhanced if communication was improved" (Lubinski et al. 1981: 46).

Nussbaum (1993) also studied the communication that occurs upon admission to a nursing home and found that the emphasis is on creating dependent relationships between the newly admitted resident and the facility (see also Heinemann, this volume). Nussbaum (1993:245) states, "The admission process framed the nursing home as an environment specially designed for those who are so physically unhealthy that all other aspects of one's life must now be ended." Upon admission, residents, particularly those with dementia, will communicate infrequently with staff and other residents. Ward et al. (2008) found that during a 12-hour observation period in a nursing home, there were only about 17.7 interactions per resident with staff, 12.9 of which were initiated by staff, and most were brief or entirely silent. Most communication focused on health care tasks (77%) and only 15% were social. Ward et al. (2008: 638) described the staff-resident interaction as "care speak," stating that verbal input by the residents was rarely required and not often elicited. In a study of residents in a Canadian facility, Dorze et al. (1994) found that residents with communication disorders are less involved in interaction than those with no communication problems.

Studies by Lubinski, Morrison and Rigrodsky (1981), and Kaakinen (1995) propose that there are unwritten but powerful rules that influence the communication occurring in long-term care settings. Examples of rules include not talking with those of the opposite gender, no gossiping or talking loudly during quiet times, no complaining, and no discussion of loneliness, dying, or oneself. Such rules contribute to reducing communication opportunities, choice of topics and partners, and overall quality of communication. Interestingly, these studies show that residents are able to articulate these rules though staff argue that there are no communicative restrictions.

The above grim portrait of communication in nursing homes is also seen in other long-term care facilities. Williams and Warren (2009:24) studied communication between residents and staff in an assisted living environment. They summarize their findings by saying that, even in this more autonomous environment, communication is problematic and similar to traditional nursing homes in its lack of opportunity to communicate and the infantilization of talk to residents. Thus, there appears to be a characteristic picture of communication impaired environments in long-term care facilities.

Assessment and Intervention

A variety of professionals are interested in creating a more positive communicative environment for older residents in long-term care facilities. Nursing staff have long had a practical and research interest in this topic. Speech-language pathologists are also interested in how individuals with whom they work can use their communication skills in a more effective and functional way. If a positive communication environment is to be achieved, however, a broad coalition of professional staff members, volunteers, and family members must be aware of their roles in creating a positive communication environment.

The question becomes how to effectively and efficiently assess the communication skills, effectiveness, and opportunities of older residents and how to create practical strategies for intervention in long-term care settings. Professionals who are likely to be involved in assessment and intervention include nursing/medical staff, speech-language pathologists, audiologists, vision specialists, activities directors, social workers and psychologists, as well as other rehabilitation specialists. Family members, personal care assistants, and volunteers can also initiate an evaluation request and offer input into the assessment and intervention process.

In the United States communication skills are routinely assessed upon admission to long-term care facilities that receive Medicare and Medicaid funding. Vision, hearing, communication, cognition, and emotional screenings are all included in the Minimum Data Set 3.0 (MDS 3.0), a standardized assessment tool promulgated by the Centers for Medicare and Medicaid (CMS) and used in all Medicare certified nursing/post-acute facilities in the United States. Ideally, objective and reliable measures of these skills are obtained in addition to resident and staff subjective appraisals of all communication modalities and sensory, cognitive, and emotional skills.

Lubinski (2010) recently presented a tool entitled "Communication Profile of Long-Term Care Resident" that can be used as a guide to evaluate each of these areas (see Appendix). The guide provides a summary of a resident's communication skills, effectiveness, and opportunities. It incorporates a four-point scale (0 to 3) similar to that used in the Communication Section on the Minimum Data Set 3.0. Evaluators are free to choose appropriate tools consistent with resident needs and cultural background to assess communication skills. The profile also alerts the assessor to the need for intervention that might include further evaluation, referral to another specialist, or direct modification.

Other tools that might be used to evaluate the communication environment of a long-term care facility include the "Communication Environment Inventory" (Lubinski 2008). This assessment provides a more in-depth analysis of the physical and social environment of nursing homes or other environments where older persons reside. Hickson et al. (2005) have also developed a tool to assess nursing home residents' communication impairments, activity limitations, and participation.

Communication Skills Intervention

Intervention begins by remediating communication skills to the highest degree possible. For example, traditional speech-language therapy is appropriate for those with communication problems related to stroke, traumatic brain injury, progressive neurological disorders such as Parkinson's disease, and other communication impairments. Goals for rehabilitation need to be functional and relevant to the daily interaction of older residents in long-term care settings. When possible, goals should focus on communication related to care and safety, but also to social interactions with caregivers, family, and friends.

Also essential is provision of communication-assistive devices such as hearing aids, assistive listening devices, communication expressive technologies, and corrective vision aids. Examples of auditory communication aids include personal hearing aids, assistive listening devices, and FM environmental technologies. Not all older persons will be candidates for personal hearing aids, and referral to an audiologist who is familiar with how to fit those with compromised cognition is important (see Kricos 2006). Vision aids include eyeglasses, magnifiers, telescopes, large print contrast materials, computer technology, closed circuit television, optical character recognition technologies, listening devices, tape recorders, radio reading services, reading machines, and time device technologies (Independent Living Aids 2010; Low Vision Aids 2010).

It is necessary not only that older residents have appropriate communication aids but also that caregivers support their use and ensure their working order. Caregivers need to understand the importance of using such aids and know how to incorporate their use. Furthermore, speech-language pathologists or others providing remediation need to educate caregivers regarding the goals of rehabilitation and how caregivers can reinforce newly improved skills in everyday interaction.

Numerous programs exist for improving the cognitive or emotional status of older residents—a topic that is too long for this paper. Professionals implementing these programs, however, should consider how critical communication is for their success. Improving cognition and emotional status encourages older residents to communicate to their potential and helps others see them as viable communication partners.

Effectiveness Intervention

Communicative effectiveness is achieved through two foci: (i) the development and use of alternative and assistive communication strategies and devices, and (ii) the education of family and professional caregivers in how to use and apply them. Both of these goals can be achieved through in-service and education programs. It has to be kept in mind, though, that such educational programs need to be frequent and offered at various times so that staff and family can easily access training.

The outcomes of education should result in staff and families being able to understand the value of communication in the life of older residents and in the provision of quality care and to use a variety of personal and environmental strategies to promote successful communication with older residents. In addition to learning about communication changes associated with normal and pathological aging, staff and family must realize their critical and reciprocal role in the communication life of older residents. They must be committed to solving difficult communication breakdowns, and their use of effective communication strategies should be reinforced. Practical strategies for in-service implementation have been discussed by Koury and Lubinski (1995).

A number of training programs have been used with nursing home staff and found effective. For example, Ripich et al. (1995) studied the outcomes of the "FOCUSED" communication skills program on the knowledge and communication satisfaction of nursing assistants who worked with residents with Alzheimer's disease. Results indicated that caregivers improved in their knowledge and use of communication strategies and reported more favorable attitudes and satisfaction when communicating with residents with Alzheimer's disease. Bryan et al. (2002) also found that their training program called "Communicate" resulted in improved self-assessments of knowledge about communication and competence concerning communication problems of older residents. Williams et al. (2003) trained nursing assistants to reduce their use of elderspeak with older residents. In addition, assistants used an emotional tone in their speech that was less controlling and more respectful (see also Williams, this volume).

McCallion et al. (1999) concluded that their "Family Visit Education Program" significantly increased caregivers' use of encouragement and that residents used fewer verbally agitated behaviors during family visits. Levy-Storms (2008) reviewed 13 studies focusing on training nursing assistants in therapeutic communication with older residents with cognitive impairment in long-term care settings. Results indicate that nursing assistants can improve their therapeutic communication especially through the use of open-ended questions, positive statements, eye contact, as well as touching and smiling. Two critical reviews of caregiver programs to improve communication with persons with Alzheimer's disease can be found in Egan et al. (2010) and Zientz et al. (2007).

Creating Opportunities for Communication

Intervention to improve the physical and social environment is also needed to complete the comprehensive approach to improving the communication life of older persons in long-term care facilities. Intervention may be implemented through design of the built environment and through in-services to staff and families to help them understand the effect of the physical and social environment on communication.

The designed physical environment must become "communication-friendly" by providing easy access to ample communication opportunities. These opportunities should reflect the interests, needs, and culture of older residents and their communication partners. Residents must also perceive that they can access people and activities that engender conversations. This may be done independently or with readily available assistance. The physical environment must also accommodate the sensory and cognitive changes associated with aging and dementia. Lubinski (2008) suggests that four elements of the physical environment should be addressed: (i) lighting and visual cues, (ii) the auditory environment, (iii) furniture arrangement, and (iv) environmental stimuli or props (Lubinski 2008: 334). Areas of the long-term environment should be available for congregate and small group activities as well as private conversations.

Enhancement of the visual environment in long-term care settings affects how well older residents will receive verbal and nonverbal information from their communication partners, safely navigate their setting, and be visually and cognitively stimulated. Visual enrichment includes increasing the amount of controllable light, particularly natural daylight, in areas where older residents congregate and communicate. Safety is also promoted through careful lighting of areas where older residents walk. An especially important visual design element is the reduction of glare by reducing shiny surfaces, the use of controllable window treatments, and the use of landscaping design to provide glare-free congregation areas in and around facilities. Fluorescent lighting should be used judiciously because flickering may increase the distractibility of residents. Older persons also respond better to some colors than others. For example, some may have difficulty perceiving pastels, blue and green tones, and low-contrast colors (O'Keefe 2006). Color also needs to be considered for its aesthetic and orientation values. Colors and textures can be used as cues to help residents orient themselves to their environment. Depth perception is also affected by the color and patterns of floor and wall surfaces. Signage should be at eye level, distinct, glare-free, consistent, and uncomplicated.

The auditory environment is critical for the transmission and reception of verbal information. Older residents with even mild hearing losses will have difficulty understanding speech when it is presented in a noisy background. Inclusion of sound absorbing surfaces in high communication areas will help reduce sound reverberations and mitigate background noise. Areas used for communal activities and personal conversations should be sound-friendly through the use of acoustical tiling, movable acoustic screens, carpeting and upholstering, and noise seals around doors and windows. Personal and FM assistive listening devices and technologies should be available in communication areas such as day and dining rooms, around the nurses' station, and other congregate areas. Attention to the sound environment does not mean eliminating all sounds as these can be stimulating, but rather reinforcing safety and orientation cues and stimulating conversations.

Furniture arrangements in both personal and congregate areas should facilitate communicative interaction. The purpose of furniture and other props in the environment is to increase socialization and stimulation. Thus, residents need to perceive the aforementioned areas as available for communication with family, friends, and staff. Seating needs to be size appropriate, safe, comfortable, and easy to get in and out of (Christenson 1990). Seating should be movable to allow access for those in wheelchairs or using walkers and also encourage easy visual and auditory access to communication partners and activities.

The environment should also contain numerous props that promote orientation, cognitive and social stimulation, safety, and aesthetics. Of critical importance for residents is their perception that they can personalize their environment with their own furniture, pictures, and the "stuff of life" that reflects their personality, interests, and history. A variety of stimulating objects such as computers, books, magazines, games, crafts, plants, and pets should be easily accessible.

Technology can also be considered part of the environment and can promote cognitive stimulation, interaction, enjoyment, and independence (Tak et al. 2007). Assistive and alternative communication options (AAC) used with residents who have expressive aphasia and motor speech disorders frequently involve high-technology devices. For other residents, technology may focus on individual computers with adaptive keyboards or voice recognition, connection to the Internet, interactive gaming, cognitive training programs, and music creation and playback. Webcams and videophones are especially good for connecting residents and families in the community (Demiris et al. 2008). Technology has even been used successfully to educate families of nursing home residents (Rosen et al. 2003). For a discussion of computer programs used in nursing homes, see the Minnesota Department of Health (2009).

Some technology is used to assist older residents who have cognitive impairments. Pollack (2005: 12) proposes that technology provides assurance about safety, helps residents compensate for impairments, and assesses their cognitive status. Activity monitoring technology includes sensors to monitor the environment and the resident. Compensation systems include navigational devices, phones, and schedule management and reminder systems.

Activities that are age appropriate and cognitively stimulating also inspire interaction. Older residents will talk about what they are doing, and the activities in which they participate should encourage interaction. While games such as bingo and musical programs are popular, it is the interaction inspired by the activity that is truly important. Other adult-like activities that stimulate interaction include debates, participation in resident government, education, political and religious discussions, physical exercise, holiday specials, senior proms, and programs designed and implemented by residents themselves. Whenever possible, activities should reflect the cultural background of the resident and include family and friends who reflect this history. Some older residents may want to contribute to chores in the residential setting or serve as communication buddies to isolated residents. Activities that are cross generational and outside this setting should be encouraged whenever possible. Staff should engage residents in conversations about their activities and reinforce their participation.

Good sources of information on the environmental design for older residents include Aging Eye (2006), Barnes, (2002), Brawley (1997), Calkins (1988), Christenson (1990), and O'Keefe (2006).

Practical Implications

This paper proposes that the communication life of older residents in long-term care settings should be a priority for residents, caregivers, and families. When older residents can communicate effectively, the quality of their care is enhanced, caregivers feel more fulfilled in their role, and most importantly, residents maximize their independence, strengthen their social connectedness, and enhance their sense of self-worth. This chapter has outlined a comprehensive tripartite model for creating a positive communication environment in which older residents can fulfill their communication needs. The model also provides a template for understanding the specific communication needs of older residents and presents practical strategies for both assessment and intervention.

The first component of this communication model focuses on assessing and remediating the receptive and expressive communication skills of older residents as well as the visual, hearing, cognitive, and emotional skills that support and influence the ability to communicate. Assessment and rehabilitation should be provided to maximize these skills to the highest level possible.

The second component of the communication model focuses on effectiveness. Older residents may need alternative and augmentative strategies or technology to help them communicate effectively. They also need communication partners, primarily staff and family, who know how to facilitate communication and repair communication breakdowns when they occur. Attention to communication partners underscores communication as a dyadic process and the importance of *both* interlocutors. Communication in-services/education should be readily and frequently available for all staff and family members. Such programs may need to be presented at non-standard times such as evenings and weekends to attract a wide audience.

The final part of the model focuses on the physical and social context in which communication occurs in long-term care settings. It is not sufficient to have adequate skills, skilled partners, and available technologies to support communication if there are only few or no opportunities that stimulate it or if the environment itself extinguishes it. Attention should be paid to how the sensory and cognitive environment supports communication, physical access to partners and activities, personalization of the environment, and technology to create and augment conversations. Older residents deserve to live in an environment that respects them, values their input, and provides plentiful, supportive, and stimulating opportunities to communicate.

Appendix

Communication Profile of Long-Term Care Resident

Name____________ Date of Evaluation____________
Reevaluation________ Facility________ Room________
Date of Admission______ DOB______ Age______ Gender______
Marital Status________ Spouse________ Family Member______
Diagnosis______ Hearing Aid______ Glasses______ Other aid______
Preferred Language______ Ambulatory______ Education______
Other:____________ Completed by____________

Communication Area	Adequacy[1]				Intervention Needed[2]
	0	1	2	3	Yes
	No Problem	Minimal Difficulty	Moderate Difficulty	Severe Difficulty	
Communication Skills					
1. Vision Aid used______	0	1	2	3	Yes______

2. Hearing Aid used_______	0	1	2	3	Yes_______
3. Receptive communication Tool used_______	0	1	2	3	Yes_______
4. Expressive communication Tool used_______	0	1	2	3	Yes_______
5. Cognition Tool used_______	0	1	2	3	Yes_______
6. Emotions Tool used_______	0	1	2	3	Yes_______
Communication Effectiveness					
7. Gets meaning across via verbal &/or nonverbal means	0	1	2	3	Yes_______
8. Uses assistive aid or alternate strategy to facilitate communication	0	1	2	3	Yes_______
9. Communication partners are communicatively skilled	0	1	2	3	Yes_______
Communication Opportunities **Physical Environment**					
10. Physical design promotes interaction	0	1	2	3	Yes_______
11. Access to activities & communication partners	0	1	2	3	Yes_______
12. Lighting adequate in communication areas	0	1	2	3	Yes_______
13. Noise control in communication areas	0	1	2	3	Yes_______
14. Private places to talk	0	1	2	3	Yes_______
15. Assistive devices promote communication	0	1	2	3	Yes_______
Psychosocial Environment					
16. Variety of activities to stimulate thinking & interaction	0	1	2	3	Yes_______
17. Communication promoted during resident care	0	1	2	3	Yes_______
18. Communication partners use adult-like speech with resident	0	1	2	3	Yes_______
19. Resident to resident talk encouraged	0	1	2	3	Yes_______
20. Communication is an important part of resident's daily life	0	1	2	3	Yes_______

Other Comments:

[1] **Adequacy Scale:** 0 = No problem that affects communication on daily basis
1 = Difficulty affects resident infrequently—less than 25% of time
2 = Difficulty affects resident frequently but not always
3 = Difficulty affects resident most of the time—75% or more of time

[2] **Intervention Needed:** Denotes that an assessment, referral to specialist, or direct modification is needed.

References

Aging Eye. (2006). *Eye Changes with Aging.* Available at http://agingeye.net/visionbasics/theaging eye.php (last accessed 25 September 2010).

AHCA (American Health Care Association). (2010). *What is Oscar Data?* www.ahcancal.org/research_data/oscar_data/Pages/WhatisOSCARData.aspx. (last accessed 25 September 2010).

ASHA (American Speech-Language and Hearing Association). (2004). *Communication Disorders in Older Americans.* www.asha.org/about/news/tipsheets/04MarchTP.htm (last accessed 13 September 2010).

Bagley, M. (1995). The challenge to independence: Severe vision and hearing loss among older adults. *American Rehabilitation* (Summer, 1995). www.thefreelibrary.com/The+challenge+to+independence%3A+severe+vision+and+hearing+loss+among . . . -a017986036 (last accessed 13 September 2010).

Barnes, S. (2002). The design of caring environments and the quality of life of older people. *Aging and Society* 22. 775–89.

Berry, P., J. Mascia & B. Steinman. (2004). Vision and hearing loss in older adults. *Care Management Journals* 5. 35–40.

Better Hearing Institute. (2004). Hearing loss going undetected in nursing homes. www.betterhearing.org/press/hearingnews/pr_nursingHomes.cfm/ (last accessed 13 September 2010).

Brawley, E. (1997). *Designing for Alzheimer's Disease.* New York: Wiley & Sons.

Bryan, K., J. Axelrod, L. Maxim & L. Jordan. (2002). Working with older people with communication difficulties; an evaluation of care worker training. *Aging and Mental Health* 6. 248–54.

Calkins, M. (1988). Design for dementia. In M. P. Calkins, *Planning Environments for the Elderly and Confused.* Owings Mills, MD: National Health.

Cassie, R. & E. Rockwell. (1994). Communication difficulties experienced by nursing home residents with a hearing loss during conversation with staff members. *Journal of Speech-Language Pathology and Audiology* 18. 127–34.

Christenson, M. (1990). *Aging in the Designed Environment.* New York: Haworth Press.

Congdon, N, B. O'Colmain, C. Klaver, R. Klein, B. Munoz, D. Friedman, J. Kempen, H. Taylor & P. Mitchell. (2004). Causes and prevalence of visual impairment among adults in the United States. *Archives of Opthalmology* 122. 477–85.

Demiris, G., D. Oliver, B. Hensel, G. Dickey, M. Ramtz & M. Skubic. (2008). Use of videophones for distant caregiving. *Journal of Gerontological Nursing* 34. 50–5.

Dorze, G., M. Julien, C. Brassard, J. Durocher & G. VeBoivin. (1994). An analysis of the communication of adult residents of a long-term care hospital as perceived by their caregivers. *International Journal of Language and Communication Disorders* 29. 241–68.

Egan, M., D. Berube, G. Racine, C. Leonard & E. Rochon. (2010). Methods to enhance verbal communication between individuals with Alzheimer's disease and formal and informal caregivers: A systematic review. *International Journal of Alzheimer's Disease* Vol. 2010. www.sage-hindawi.com/journals/ijad/2010/906818.html (last accessed 13 September 2010).

Garahan, M., J. Walter, M. Houghton, W. Tisdale & C. Runge. (1992). Hearing loss prevalence and management in nursing home residents. *Journal of the American Geriatrics Society* 40. 130–4.

Garcia, L. & J. B. Orange. (1996). The analysis of conversation skills of older adults: Current research and clinical approaches. *Journal of Speech-Language Pathology and Audiology* 20. 326–32.

Gold, M., L. Lightfoot & T. Hnath-Chosolm. (1996). Hearing loss in a memory disorders clinic: A specially vulnerable population. *Archives of Neurology* 53. 922–8.

Grainger, K. (2004). Communication and the institutionalized elderly. In J. F. Nussbaum and J. Coupland (eds), *Handbook of Communication and Aging Research*, 2nd edn, 479–97. Mahwah, NJ. and London: Laurence Erlbaum Associates.

Hickson, L., L. Worrall, J. Wilson, C. Tilse & D. Setterlund. (2005). Evaluating communication for resident participation in an aged care facility. *International Journal of Speech-Language Pathology* 7. 245–57.

Independent Living Aids. (2010). www.independentliving.com

Jones, R., E. Marcantonio & T. Rabinowitz. (2005). Prevalence and correlates of recognized depression in U.S. nursing homes. *Journal of the American Geriatrics Society* 51. 1404–9.

Jongenelis, K., A. Pot, A. Eisses, A. Beekman, H. Kluiter & M. Ribbe. (2004). Prevalence and risk indicators of depression in elderly nursing home patients: The AGED study. *Journal of Affective Disorders* 83. 135–42.

Kaakinen, J. (1995). Talking among elderly nursing home residents. *Topics in Language Disorders* 15. 36–46.

Koury, L. & R. Lubinski. (1995). Effective inservice-training for staff working with communication-impaired patients. In R. Lubinski (ed.), *Dementia and Communication*, 279–91. Clifton Park, New York: Delmar Learning.

Krauss, N. & B. Altman. (1996). *Research Findings #5: Characteristics of Nursing Home Residents.* Rockville, MD: U.S. Department of Health & Human Services. www.meps.ahrq.gov/mepsweb/data_files/publications/rf5/rf5.shtml (last accessed 13 September 2010).

Kricos, P. (2006). Audiologic management of older adults with hearing loss and compromised cognitive/psychoacoustic auditory processing abilities. *Trends in Amplification* 10. 1–28.

Levy-Storms, L. (2008). Therapeutic communication training in long-term care institutions: Recommendations for future research. *Patient Education and Counseling* 73. 8–21.

Lighthouse International. (2006). Dual sensory impairment among the elderly. Overview. www.lighthouse.org (last accessed 13 September 2010).

Low Vision Aids. (2010). http://lowvision.org. (last accessed 25 September 2010)

Lubinski, R. (2008). Environmental approach to aphasia. In R. Chapey (ed.), *Language Intervention Strategies in Aphasia and Related Neurogenic Communication Disorders*, 319–48. Philadelphia: Wolters Kluwer.

—(2010). *A Model for Communication Intervention with the Elderly.* Paper presented at the 28th World Congress of the International Association of Logopedics and Phoniatrics, Athens, Greece, 22–6 August, 2010.

Lubinski, R., Morrison, E. & S. Rigrodsky. (1981). Perception of spoken communication by elderly chronically ill patients in an institutional setting. *Journal of Speech and Hearing Disorders* 46. 405–12.

Matthews, F. & T. Dening. (2002). Prevalence of dementia in institutional care. *Lancet* 36. 225–8.

McCallion, P., R. Tosesland & K. Freeman. (1999). An evaluation of a family visit education program. *Journal of the American Geriatrics Society* 47. 203–14.

Minnesota Department of Health. (2009). *Summary Evaluation of Nursing Home Technology Pilot Projects, Including Successes, Challenges and Lessons Learned.* www.careproviders.org/members/2009/NHTechnologyPilotGrantProjectEvalSummaryJune09.pdf (last accessed 13 September 2010).

National Eye Institute. (2010). *Prevalence of Cataract, Age-related Macular Degeneration, and Open-angle Glaucoma Among Adults 40 Years and Older in the United States.* www.nei.nih.gov/eyedata/pbd_tables.asp (last accessed 13 September 2010).

Nussbaum, J. (1993). The communicative impact of institutionalization for the elderly: The admissions process. *Journal of Aging Studies* 7. 237–46.

O'Keefe, J. (2006). *Creating a Senior Friendly Physical Environment in our Hospitals.* Ottawa, Canada: Regional Geriatric Assessment Program of Ottawa.

Orange, J. B. & B. Purves. (1996). Conversational discourse and cognitive impairment: Implications for Alzheimer's disease. *Journal of Speech-Language Pathology and Audiology* 20. 139–54.

Orr, A. (1997). Assistive technologies for older persons who are visually impaired. In R. Lubinski and J. Higginbotham (Eds) *Communication Technologies for the Elderly: Vision, Hearing and Speech*, 171–201. San Diego: Singular Press.

Pollack, M. (2005). Intelligent technology for an aging population. *AI Magazine* (Summer 2005). 9–24.

Resnick, H., B. Fries & L. Verbrugger. (1997). Windows to their world: The effect of sensory impairments on social engagement and activity time in nursing home residents. *The Journals of Gerontology Series B Psychological Sciences and Social Sciences* 52. 135–44.

Ripich, D., M. Wykle & S. Niles. (1995). Alzheimer's disease caregivers: The FOCUSED program. *Geriatric Nursing* 16. 15–19.

Rosen, J., V. Mittal, B. Mulsant, H. Degenholtz, N. Castle & D. Fox. (2003). Educating the families of nursing home residents: A pilot study using a computer-based system. *Journal of the American Medical Directors Association* 4. 128–34.

Rovner, B., P. German, J. Broadhead, R. Morris, L. Brout, J. Blaustein & M. Folstein. (1990). The prevalence and management of dementia and other psychiatric disorders. *International Psychogeriatrics* 2. 13–24.

Senior Journal. (2009). *Nine Trends in Global Aging Present Challenges.* http://seniorjournal.com/.NEWS/SeniorStats/2007/7–03-16-NineTrends.htm.(last accessed 25 September 2010).

Stone, R. (2000). *Long-term Care for the Elderly with Disabilities. Current Policy, Emerging Trends, and Implications for the Twenty-first Century* (Milbank reports, August 2000) New York: Milbank Memorial Fund. www.milbank.org/reports/0008stone/LongTermCare_Mech5.pdf (last accessed 13 September 2010).

Tak, S., C. Beck & E. McMahon. (2007). Computer and internet access for long-term care residents. *Journal of Gerontological Nursing* 33. 32–40.

Tielsch, J., J. Javitt, A. Coleman, J. Katz & A. Sommer. (1995). The prevalence of blindness and visual impairment among nursing home residents in Baltimore. *New England Journal of Medicine* 332. 1205–9.

Uhlmann, R., E. Larson, T. Rees, T. Koepsell & L. Duckert. (1989). Relationship of hearing impairment to dementia and cognitive dysfunction in older adults. *Journal of the American Medical Association* 261. 1916–19.

Vision Help. (2010). www.visionhelp.com. (last accessed 25 September 2010).

Wagenaar, D., C. Colenda, M. Kreft, J. Sawade, J. Gardiner & E. Poverejan. (2003). Treating depression in nursing homes: Practice guidelines in the real world. *Journal of the American Osteopathic Association* 103. 465–9.

Ward, R., A. Vass, N. Aggarwal, C. Garfield & B. Cybyk. (2008). A different story: Exploring patterns of communication in residential dementia care. *Aging and Society* 28. 629–51.

Williams, K., S. Kemper & M. Hummert. (2003). Improving nursing home communication: An intervention to reduce elderspeak. *Gerontologist* 43. 242–7.

Williams, K. & C. Warren. (2009). Communication in assisted living. *Journal of Aging Studies* 23. 24–36.

Worrall, L. & L. Hickson. (2003). *Communication Disability in Aging.* Clifton Park, New York: Thomson Delmar Learning.

Worrall, L., L. Hickson & B. Dodd. (1993). Screening for communication impairment in nursing homes. *Australian Journal of Human Communication Disorders* 21. 53–64.

Zientz, J., A. Rackley, S. Chapman, T. Hopper., N. Mahendra, E. Kim & S. Cleary. (2007). Evidence-based practice recommendations for dementia: Educating caregivers on Alzheimer's disease and training communication strategies. *Journal of Medical Speech-Language Pathology* 15. iiii–ixiv.

Chapter 4

Care of People with Alzheimer's Disease in New Zealand: Supporting the Telling of Life Stories

Margaret Maclagan and Annabel Grant

Introduction

In this chapter we consider the care of older people with Alzheimer's disease in New Zealand. We will first outline New Zealand's demographics before turning to areas that relate specifically to old people. After describing the types of facilities and typical care available in New Zealand, we will report on two studies that use reminiscence to examine communication with people with Alzheimer's disease. We finish with suggestions for clinical practitioners.

New Zealand Demographics

New Zealand has a population of approximately 4,365,000 (Department of Statistics 2010a). It is projected to pass 5 million in the mid-2020s and reach 5.75 million by 2061. The population is rapidly aging. Those aged 65+ are projected to increase from 550,000 in 2009 to 1 million in the late 2020s, and will then exceed the number of children aged 0–14 years. One in five New Zealanders will be aged 65+ by 2031, compared with one in eight in 2009 (Department of Statistics 2010b). In the 2006 census, approximately 73% of the population identified themselves as New Zealand or European (usually called *Pakeha*), 14% as Maori, 7% as Pacific Islanders (usually called *Pasifika*) and 6% as Asian (Department of Statistics 2009). The Pakeha group is clearly the largest group, but the Maori, Pasifika, and Chinese groups are currently growing much faster than the Pakeha group.

Table 4.1. Prevalence of dementia by age group

Age Group	Prevalence
All people 65+	7.7%
65–74	3.8%
75–79	6.4%
80–84	11.0%
85–89	23.6%
90+	40.4%

Data sourced from: Ministry of Health (1997).

As the population ages, so the number of people with dementia increases. The non-profit organization Alzheimer's New Zealand Incorporated (ANZI 2008) estimates that in 2008, 40,746 New Zealanders had dementia. This figure is projected to increase to 74,821 by 2026. Current indications of the prevalence of dementia across the population are that 1,483 (3.6%) are Maori, 1,227 (3.0%) are Asian, 683 (1.7%) are Pacific Islanders, and 37,790 (92.7%) are European or other. Clearly, dementia disproportionately affects the Pakeha group, with proportionately fewer coming from the other groups. More women (60.2%) than men (39.8%) are estimated to have dementia, and the number rises across the age groups (see Table 4.1). There were an estimated 12,333 new cases of Alzheimer's disease in New Zealand in 2008. It is estimated that 60% of all people currently in residential care (21,000 people) have dementia. This figure is projected to be 31,000 by 2020, and almost 76,000 by 2050.

Care in New Zealand

Types of Care

Over the last ten to fifteen years the number of Retirement villages in New Zealand has increased greatly (Boyd et al. 2009). Retirement villages cater for people who prefer independent living. Not all of them include facilities for residential care, but those that do must be licensed by the Ministry of Health. If people need a greater level of care, they move into a rest home. Those with dementia will eventually move to a specialist dementia care rest home, which will have a secure facility, and possibly then to a long-stay hospital.

The current emphasis in New Zealand health politics is to maintain people in their own home for as long as possible. Boyd et al. (2009: 1) emphasize a lack of facilities for older persons, noting that "Aged residential care bed numbers have increased by only 3% in the last 20 years in Auckland, despite a 43% increase in the population over the age of 65 years." As more people move into residential care, so the importance of skilled caregivers increases.[1]

Implications of the Increasing Numbers of Old People in New Zealand

The predicted increase in dementia will have implications for facility staffing, where, historically, staff receive low pay and suffer high turnover rates (Ministry of Health 2002a). Caregivers generally have relatively low levels of education and experience many job-related time pressures (Ministry of Health 2004). In addition there is an increasing reliance on immigrant workers for caregiving in New Zealand. The vast majority of those who care for old people are female. Badkar and her colleagues (2009) indicate that in 1991 only 19% of women employed as caregivers for the elderly were born overseas; by 2006 this number had risen to 24%. In 2003 most overseas-born caregivers came from the United Kingdom and thus were presumably fluent in English. By 2008 the number of overseas-born caregivers had increased greatly, with women from the Philippines forming 52% of those born overseas. In addition, the number of caregivers from Fiji and other Polynesian countries increased over this time, producing an increase in the number of caregivers with limited English language proficiency.

Residential care challenges include "increasing ongoing training for all care staff in dementia-specific and quality person-centered care principles" (ANZI 2008). Person-centered care emphasizes valuing people, treating them as individuals, considering the other person's perspective, and promoting a positive social environment leading to well-being (Brooker 2004). Working with people with dementia is demanding and stressful, and caregivers have varying levels of knowledge and skill. Generic training programs may not be effective for removing the communication barriers experienced by individuals with dementia and may therefore fail to meet the standards expected of adequate person-centered care.

At present there are insufficient numbers of people working in the area of mental health of older people and especially in the area of dementia. The Ministry of Health first noted this need in its Health of Older People Strategy report (Ministry of Health 2002b) and recommended that improved training programs be made available in order to deliver high quality residential care. New Zealand research has identified that support workers want time and remuneration for training attendance, and better recognition of training completion, as well as more opportunities for career progression (Jorgensen et al. 2009; Ministry of Health 2004).

Caregiver training is not mandatory in New Zealand and it is "estimated that fewer than half of all caregivers have a vocational qualification. Low pay and lack of a career path also make recruitment and retention difficult" (Wilson 2009). However, there is a national service contract for Age Related Residential Care (ARRC) between providers and District Health Boards. Currently, it is mandatory for all staff working in specialist dementia units in New Zealand to achieve credits in four unit standards within 12 months of commencing employment. These include demonstrating knowledge of the effects of dementia and how to manage these, as well as person-centered care of and communication with a person living with dementia (see, e.g., Careerforce 2008).

The New Zealand Ministry of Health recommends that person-centered principles should be integrated into training for dementia care staff:

> Training programmes should be designed to facilitate a person-centered approach to care and service delivery, which recognizes the uniqueness of the person with dementia. More attention should be focused on the social, psychological and communication needs of residents such as reminiscence therapy, validation therapy and reality orientation. (Ministry of Health 2002a:38)

A recent Alzheimer's New Zealand report recommended improving education and support for residential care staff by increasing quality dementia-specific programs based on person-centered principles. To achieve this it is suggested that care staff need an in-depth personalized knowledge of the individual's history, family connections and values (ANZI 2008). Under the umbrella of person-centered care, analysis of the conversational interactions between the person with dementia and their caregiver becomes increasingly relevant.

Language in Dementia

One of the first signs of dementia is loss of recent memory coupled with repeated questions, alongside problems expressing and understanding language (Wayne and Segal 2009).[2] Language problems increase as Alzheimer's disease progresses. Semantics are compromised early so that language becomes relatively "content-less" (Chertkow and Bub 1990; Nicolas et al. 1986), but syntax, phonology, and pragmatics are left relatively intact (Dijkstra et al. 2004; Kempler et al. 1998; Ulatowska et al. 1988). In the late stages of the disease, people are usually no longer able or willing to hold a conversation, but they will often respond appropriately to greetings or attempt to answer simple questions (Temple et al.1999). Pauses become considerably longer, and it can be difficult for the conversational partner to assess whether the person with Alzheimer's disease has finished what they were saying or whether they are still processing their turn (Davis and Maclagan 2009). In addition, people in later stages of Alzheimer's disease tend to lose the thread of any story they are telling (Ash et al. 2007; Davis and Maclagan 2009; Boyd and Smith, this volume). While intervention cannot prevent the ongoing decline of language, skilled facilitation can help maintain the interactional skills of a person with Alzheimer's disease for as long as possible.

Reminiscence

One of the consequences of the cognitive-communication difficulties experienced by people with dementia is that they are unable to reminisce and retell their life stories in a coherent manner (Baldwin 2006). Given that reminiscence is part of the normal psychological development of older adults, with benefits for successful aging, it is important to consider the impact dementia may have on the ability to reminisce and specifically to maintain self-identity (Wong and Watt 1991). Rather than being an "aimless wandering of the mind," reminiscence is part of a wider process of reviewing one's life, a process which occurs in all older people, including those who are "adequately functioning" (Butler 1963). People with dementia must be able to continue to talk about their lives because it is this narrative or self-story that preserves their identity. A good life story has been described as one that has the properties of coherence, structure (beginning, middle and end), assimilation and interpretation of events, and truthfulness (Coleman 1999). People with dementia experience a loss of cohesion and coherence in their discourse, and this, together with memory loss, makes it difficult to organize narratives of personal history (Leichtman et al. 2003).

Contrary to views on dementia presented in both popular and healthcare literature, studies are emerging which offer evidence that self-identity is maintained and preserved even in the latter stages of dementia (Fazio and Mitchell 2009; Surr 2006; Ryan and Schindel Martin, this volume). Self-identity can be preserved in people with dementia by virtue of the caregiver's continued belief that the person still exists in self and mind, even when the body's functions become solely vegetative (Gubrium 2005). Kitwood (1997) talks about identity being "held in place", by virtue of knowledge of the life story of the person with dementia when that person is unable to tell their story (see also Ulatowska and Bond Chapman 1991). Caregivers can choose to accept the inaccuracies inherent in the stories of people with dementia and view these as an extension of a normal process of imperfect remembering (Singer and Blagov 2004). Engaging in reminiscence can delay the communication breakdown between people with dementia and others. As memory fails, the life story or narrative is gradually handed over to caregivers for retelling.

A number of studies have investigated memory aids for people with dementia, which often include life story information, with the aim of solving issues caused by memory loss. Memory wallets for enhancing communication between people with dementia and their family members were first introduced by Bourgeois (1990). These wallets contained facts about the person in the categories "my day," "myself," and "my life." A subsequent study by Bourgeois (1993) found that the wallets increased the number of factual statements and decreased the number of erroneous or ambiguous utterances made by the participants. After the aid was provided, participants took longer and more frequent conversational turns, showing improved quality of conversation between dyads (two people with dementia). These memory aids were presented initially as wallets. Today, they are usually books or even electronic resources (Davis et al., in press). A single case study of a person with moderate to severe dementia found that in conversations in which the memory book was utilized by the caregiver, more topics were covered and in more detail (Spilkin and Bethlehem 2003). Individuals with severe dementia also benefit, making more on-topic statements when a memory book is used (Andrews-Salvia et al. 2003). However, the results of these studies were obtained in a highly structured environment with the researcher providing cues and it is unclear whether similar improvements would be found in a more natural environment.

The following presents two studies that used reminiscence with people with dementia in considerably less structured and more natural ways. A focus of both studies was to maintain or increase the amount of reminiscence that the participants were able to engage in when conversing with a familiar person, and thus help them maintain their sense of self.

Outline of the Studies

We report first on the study carried out by Grant, the second author of this chapter. The study comprised two conversations between each of three dyads consisting of a person with Alzheimer's disease (Evie, George, May) and his or her regular caregiver. In each conversation the caregivers were asked to talk to their partners about their partners' lives. The first conversation provided a baseline for the conversational competence of the participants with dementia. Between the first and second conversations, the researcher developed memory books for the participants and the caregiver used these books in the

Table 4.2. Participants in the two reported studies

	Study 1			Study 2
	Evie	**George**	**May**	**Doreen**
Age	73	82	82	84
Sex	F	M	F	F
MMSE	17	18	8	–

Note: All participant names have been changed to preserve anonymity. MMSE stands for Mini Mental State Examination (see Folstein et al. 1975), an examination that is used to gauge the severity of cognitive impairment. The numbers indicate moderate impairment for Evie and George, and severe impairment for May.

second conversations. The time between the first and second conversations in Study 1 varied from three to six months.

The second study we report on was carried out by Maclagan, the first author of this chapter. It consisted of conversations every two weeks between a trained research assistant and a woman (Doreen), who was in the early to moderate stages of Alzheimer's disease. The interviewer in Study 2 was instructed to start her interaction by finding out what she could about Doreen's life history. Doreen had family photograph albums and these were used as resources. Table 4.2 presents the demographics for the participants reported on here.

Methodology

The conversations in Study 1 were recorded on video; the conversations in Study 2 were recorded as audio.[3] All conversations were then transcribed with all hesitations included and no tidying. For Study 2, pauses were measured using Praat acoustic analysis software (Boersma and Weenink 2009).

To develop the memory books for Study 1, background biographical information was gathered from the older person and family member/proxy using a standard form (Bourgeois 2007). Photos were chosen by a family member. The researcher scanned the photos, and then inserted them into a word-processed document along with the background information to cover key aspects of the person's life story, such as family, significant events, and hobbies. An individualized memory book was produced for each older person containing the photographs, interspersed with captions and simple short sentences that elaborated on the pictures or aspects of the individual's life story. A first draft was shown to the family member/proxy to confirm the information was correct and to approve the layout. The draft was also shown to the older person for their approval, and photos that appeared to cause distress were excluded.

In keeping with the busy schedules at most residential care facilities, the caregivers were given minimal instruction in how to use the memory books. Training with the memory book consisted of a brief individualized session (30–45 minutes) that covered the use of the memory book and how to improve conversations with the older person. The session was delivered by a qualified speech and language pathologist (the second author of this chapter). Training content was chosen based on the skills observed in the videotaped first conversation samples as measured by the "Strategies to improve communication checklist" (Jordan et al. 2000) and a conversation analysis of those samples, as well as on answers provided by the caregiver to a knowledge and attitudes questionnaire (Jordan et al. 2000). The content of the training included some general principles, but predominantly focused on providing specific individualized advice based not only on the caregiver's performance, but also on the conversation skills demonstrated by the older person. The second author of this chapter used the video and/or transcription of the original conversation to illustrate key points, positively reinforcing the strategies that the caregiver used to help the conversation, such as speaking at an appropriate rate and volume. The individualized advice was framed using "FOCUSED" (Face-to-face, Orientation, Continuity, Unsticking, Structure, Exchanges, and Direct), a set of strategies to maintain communication (see Ripich, Wykle and Niles 1995). Handouts documenting all the strategies discussed in the training session were provided.

Study 1

Evie was a 72-year-old female who had been living in residential care for two months. Evie's caregiver Janet was employed privately by the family for her companionship, and had worked with Evie prior to her admission into residential care. Janet visited Evie two or three times a week for conversations and trips out, as well as undertaking recreational activities with all the other residents in the facility. In the first conversation, Janet interpreted the request to talk to Evie about her life by asking Evie questions. Evie spent the first three minutes attempting to answer questions about specific details, such as how old she was when she got married, how old she was now, and how old she was when she had her son. Janet already knew the answers to these questions and often supplied them when Evie was unable to, as shown in Extract (1). However, this was not a particularly helpful form of interaction for Evie because it highlighted her difficulty in accessing precise details in response to questions. (Transcript conventions are listed in the Appendix).

(1) Evie, Conversation 1 (13 October 2008)

E: . . . yes thirty-two when I got [married*
J: [and how old* are you now?
E: oh ha you know you forget your birthday (.) I mean you don't deliberately think ur I'm old every time all the time um no I'm now what am I if I'm August I was August the eighth so I must be about um (0.3) August (1.0) I must be somewhere about August would be August the tenth or twelfth I don't know (.) I have a [(xxx)*
J: [It was the* eighth you were born
E: I was born
J: so how old are you now?
E: so that would be I'd have to have another (xxx) I'd be oh I would think around about August the twelfth (3.0) eight *((counting under her breath using fingers))*
J: go on darling it's alright *((escorting another resident from room))* you're seventy-one Evie
E: what do you have to remind me for *((laughs))*
J: and so you got married when you were thirty-three
E: umm
J: and Luke
E: um no not quite thirty-three but I yeah I'm what did you say yeah I'm what did you say
J: you're seventy-one

E: seventy-one right yes
J: and when did you have Luke?
E: um I had Luke now if (.) I was thirty something when Luke was born thirty-seven was I (.) what how old is Luke now?
J: thirty-three
E: thirty-three and I'm [seventy-one *
J: [seventy-one *
E: thirty-three and seventy-one thirty-three seventy-one so um (.) thirty-three and seventy-one so I had Luke in my late thirties would that be right?
J: that's right and have you got any other children?
E: no never had (.) never

In the second conversation, Evie responded to the presence of the memory book by reading aloud many of the photo captions and supplementing her reading with additional information. The number of novel reminiscence statements decreased slightly in the second conversation, but the total number of reminiscence statements improved markedly from 26 to 52. Evie described photos of herself and her siblings, and used the memory book to move on to the topics of nurse training and then to her sister's wedding. She was able to elaborate on both new topics, adding reminiscence statements. The memory book allowed Evie to initiate more topics in the conversation (marked by →).

(2) Evie, Conversation 2 (5 March 2009)
(Italics indicate material read from the memory book.)

E: yes we all had curly hair and I don't know why that was cause Mum didn't (1.0) *we moved to Howick in Auckland in late 1940's* and *I went to St Cecelia's College* (.) *I always wanted to be a nurse and did my training at*
→ *Auckland Public Hospital* (.) what a grim place there
J: was it grim when you were [there*?
E: [no* we had a lot of fun you know and friends you make friends and that sort of thing (.) yes (.) no I never
→ thought of it as grim funnily enough (1.0) *this is my sister Susan's wedding* (.) *she was the first one to marry*
J: I bet that was a lovely day
→ E: yes it was (.) we had <u>red</u> dresses
J: red?

E: red dresses (.) and they had a straightish skirt at the front and a big (.) a founce a flounce at the back with a big bow
J: lovely

The second participant in Study 1, George, was an 80-year-old man who had been living in residential care for three months. He was able to talk about his work history, and where he grew up, as well as about his hobbies, marriage, and family, saying: "I can tell stories and yarns like you've never heard in your life". George's caregiver Lia was Tongan and English was her second language. In the first conversation (Extract (3)), Lia asked George a number of questions that taxed his memory. More positively, she also abandoned her line of questioning and followed what George seemed to be answering (marked by → in Extract (3)).

(3) George, Conversation 1 (19 February 2009): Lia is asking questions

L: how many vehicle have you got
G: how many do you mean of of records speed records for doing packing (.) oh I can't remember long time ago
L: I mean vehicle
G: eh?
L: how many car have you got?
G: now? we've got two three four five how many in a young family (.) youngest one
→ L: how many son have you got George?
G: we've got five six children
L: mmm altogether?
G: altogether
L: but how many daughter
G: how many daughters though oh f(xxx) four five bout five daughters fou=
L: and one son
G: no two sons
L: two sons
G: yeah

In the second conversation with the memory book, George and Lia spent longer on the topic of George's life. Lia initially used the book to comment on George's gardening, but quickly reverted to asking questions. This suggests that the minimal training had not been sufficient to overcome her natural interactional style (Extract (4)). George's responses to her questions about his sons demonstrate that he could still provide information (marked by →).

(4) George, Conversation 2 (14 May 2009): Lia is still asking questions

L: do you enjoy fishing rugby
G: oh yeah I played rugby league
L: and doing gardening that's why you do the garden outside
G: yeah
L: it's really good (.) and how many bro ah sorry how many son have you got George?
G: how many=
L: son (.) how many son have you got
G: what do you mean how many workers
L: how many son es [o en*
→ G: [sons* (.) I've got two coming along now they're developing coming into it (.) one's a farmer by trade and the other one is very keen on the accounting and ah he's very good so that-
L: is that the one he coming on (.) on Tuesday for your birthday
G: yeah (.) so those things come out easy
L: oh very happy

Extracts (3) and (4) show that if Lia had used the information in the memory book to start a topic, George would probably have been able to stay on topic for longer.

The third participant in Study 1, was an 83-year-old woman called May who had been living in residential care for about one year. Susan, a South African European, was May's designated caregiver and had known May for eight months. Initially, as is evident in Extract (5), Susan used questions and comments when talking with May about her life.

(5) May, Conversation 1 (16 December 2008)

S: aha (.) so did you have a farm or did you stay in town?
M: a farm
S: a farm (1.0) and what animals did you have on the farm?

M: (4.0) what was the normal cow what's the normal cows you have like we've got them here
S: cows? (.) and did you ever go horse riding?
M: um oh we rode our horses a lot
S: aah were you fond of horses (.) did you love riding the horses?
M: oh well it used to take us to the trees and then come back and knock us off
S: oh and you had to walk back
M: yeah *((laughs))*
S: that wasn't so good hey
M: yeah that's what she did (.) shrewd old thing
S: ohh and did you have any brothers?
M: and one brother

There were six months between the first and second conversations with May, and her conversational skills had deteriorated in the interval. There was a marked decrease in the number of reminiscence statements made by May in the second conversation, as can be seen in Extract (6). Susan had the memory book to introduce topics about which she now had details. When May was not able to recall her daughter's name (marked by →), Susan used these details to ask yes/no questions that May could answer successfully (marked by ⇒). Even though May could answer the yes/no questions, she often used minimal turns such as "yeah" without adding any new information.

(6) May, Conversation 2 (9 June 2009)

S: and you got one daughter and what's her name (3.0)
→ M: ah Lau no not Laura um (5.0) Laura that (.) I know (.) I know that's her name Laura (.) and she had um (.) I think she had some of these things quite a few of them I think at one stage
S: your daughter's name was Anne
M: yeah
⇒ S: and she had two beautiful daughters (.) Laura and Cathy
M: yeah
⇒ S: do you remember Laura and Cathy?
M: yes
S: and two little twins
M: that's right

Study 1: Summary

Even though the caregivers could have made greater use of the memory books, the participants still made more reminiscence statements in the second conversations. They also made more new statements that were relevant to the conversational topic, and George and May in particular made fewer off-topic statements. Table 4.3 shows the numbers of reminiscence statements and new on-topic statements in the first and second conversations for the three participants in Study 1.

Evie made the greatest gains in both total reminiscence statements and new on-topic statements from conversation 1 to conversation 2, which were both of the same length. The second conversations with both George and May, on the other hand, were considerably longer than the first ones, possibly because the memory books gave the caregivers a framework for the conversation.

In the case of George, the increased numbers of reminiscence statements and new on-topic statements in the second conversation are potentially misleading because the second conversation lasted longer. However, the numbers of statements per minute indicate that there was a genuine increase in the second conversation. Furthermore, George used hardly any off-topic utterances in conversation 2, where off-topic comments were frequent in conversation 1. Extract (7) gives an example of the type of off-topic utterances in the first conversation.

Table 4.3. Numbers of reminiscence statements and new on-topic statements in conversations 1 and 2 for the three participants in Study 1

	Participant	**Conversation 1**			**Conversation 2**		
		Length in min.	**#**	**# per minute**	**Length in min.**	**#**	**# per minute**
Total reminiscence statements	*Evie:*	10:00	26	2.6	10:00	52	5.2
	George:	9:50	37	3.7	11:30	56	4.6
	May:	11:20	55	4.9	15:20	30	2.0
New on-topic statements	*Evie:*	10:00	73	7.3	10:00	110	11.0
	George:	9:50	95	9.5	11:30	118	10.3
	May:	11:20	86	7.6	15:20	118	7.7

(7) George, Conversation 1: Off-topic utterances from George

G: down in Hastings we had down there a guys down there but it's just it's still put up or shut up you know you've got to really (.) it's all very well saying you know well I've got a bed and all this and that but does it work is it <u>warm</u> enough (.) my wife just bought me two different rugs yesterday

L: oh that's good

In this first conversation with George, Lia has been asking him about the wine companies he used to work for. She is trying to remember a name, and although George supplies several names, he does not find the one Lia is thinking of. George has been talking about the town where he worked, Hastings, but now gives up trying to remember wine company names and launches into off-topic utterances. Then, after a brief pause, he starts a new topic, which Lia follows up on.

May's language had deteriorated more than the others' between the first and second conversations. Although she produced fewer reminiscence statements in the second interview—at least partly because Susan provided more information with which May simply agreed as seen in Extract (6)—her total number of new on-topic statements, and the number of new statements per minute, increased slightly. Furthermore, in conversation 2, she only once deviated into her favorite topic of her first workplace.

Study 2

At the start of Study 2, Doreen had just moved into a one-bedroom unit in the assisted living section of a residential care facility. On the first visit, Sara, the interviewer, did not know any details about Doreen's life. With the help of her photograph album, Doreen was able to provide considerable detail about her life. The photograph album was not a specially constructed memory book, but one that had been in Doreen's family for some time. At that time Doreen was still in the relatively early stages of Alzheimer's disease and did not need a specific memory book. By the time Sara ceased interviewing her two years later, Doreen was able to provide considerably less spontaneous information. However, because Sara had seen her approximately every two weeks over that time, Sara knew enough to be able to help retell Doreen's story and so help to hold her identity in place (Kitwood 1997). When Sara started interviewing her, Doreen was still able to care for herself. Study 2 therefore differs from Study 1 in that Sara was a regular visitor rather than a regular caregiver. However, Sara also was a trained speech and language pathologist, who was experienced in interacting with older people and also acted as an on-call caregiver in several dementia facilities within Christchurch. It was her speech-language pathology training that allowed her to make the most of her interactions with Doreen.

Extract (8) comes from the first conversation between Sara and Doreen. Doreen is able to provide details of typical family Christmas celebrations when she was younger, as well as tell Sara what she did just over a month earlier. Because Christmas is in the summer in the southern hemisphere, a barbecue is a common way for families to celebrate it. Particularly noteworthy in this extract is the length of some of Doreen's turns (marked by →) and that she does not use any pauses longer than one second. Nor does Sara have to leave long pauses to give Doreen time to respond. Rather, Doreen appropriately overlaps Sara to comment or answer questions (marked by ⇒). Similar features can be seen in Extract (9) from the second interview two weeks later when Doreen gives details about her early schooling. In extract (9) there is one appropriate longer pause in the second highlighted utterance, in which Doreen continues her turn into the new topic of high school. Because we focused on relatively long pauses in the analysis from the second study, we used dashes to indicate pause length rather than precise timings (Crystal and Davy 1969, Gordon et al. 2007). The significant point is the occurrence of pauses longer than one or two seconds, not their precise timing.

(8) Doreen interviewed by Sara, Interview 1 (8 February 2007)

S: yep - I think we'll just have - I can sort that out when I get back *((laughs))* so you had Christmas on the farm

D: sometimes yes <yep> ah - or sometimes I - go we'd go to - my sister in law's one year and then she'd come to us the next you know - we did it that was different - different family
S: yep
D: - smaller I mean the - my husband was one of ten so
S: goodness *((laughs))*
D: uh - we didn't all get together I mean [(xxx)*
S: [you wouldn't* fit
D: no you just got - together with the ones that you lived closest to - and uh - had time together -
S: yep - mmmmm - it's quite good to take turns you can share the
→ D: yes oh well we always used to take something so - <yeah> now we have - last Chr~ year we have Christmas all together and we all took something and - just had it - sort of - barbeque style and buffet style out doors you know <yep> - mmmm
S: that's always [nice*
⇒ D: [that was* quite nice -
S: was it a good day? [here?*
⇒ D: [yes* yes it was quite nice mmmmm
S: that's good - yeah - I was i~ Blenheim at home for Christmas
D: oh yeah - mmm - oh yes it's nice to be - home with your family at Christmas [time*
S: [it is* <mmhmm> it's definitely a family time isn't [it*
⇒ D: [it* is yes

(9) Doreen interviewed by Sara, Interview 2 (21 February 2007)

S: mmm where did you go to school? -
D: well the fir~ early years up to ten I went to Timaru West school
S: mmhmm
→ D: and then when we shifted ah I went to Doylston school a little - country school - only ah two teacher school
S: oh wow *((laughs))*
→ D: *((laughs))* um - for about two years - for form one and two - - and when I went to high school I used to catch the train everyday at - Doylston and travel to Christchurch to - to Technical College
S: oh okay
D: hmm

In Extract (10) from the thirtieth interview, which was recorded 22 months after Extract (8), Sara again asks Doreen about earlier family Christmas celebrations; and in Extract (11) from the same interview she asks Doreen about what she is planning to do this year. It is immediately obvious that there are more longer pauses. To emphasize this, the extracts are presented with the pauses appearing at the beginning of a line. Compared with 22 months earlier, Doreen now has pauses over one second long within her turns (lines 5, 8, 11, 19, and 25 in Extract (10) and line 12 in Extract (11), all marked by →), and Sara leaves longer pauses before she speaks. After pauses of over two seconds, where Sara expects Doreen to make a response (lines 6 and 14 in Extract (11), marked by ⇒), Sara continues with her turn.

(10) Doreen interviewed by Sara, Interview 30 (19 November 2008)

1 S: mmm
2 -- when you were younger what did your family do for
3 Christmas?
4 D: - oh well just had a family Christmas usually just
→ 5 -- our family
6 S: - mmm hmm
7 D: - once I got married it was a bit different
→ 8 -- used to do year about or
9 - er (.) have
10 - dinner with one (.) tea with the other or <uh huh> something
→ 11 -- usually worked out all right
12 S: - yup
13 -- to fit it all in
14 - <mm> because your husband he came from a large family
15 didn't he?
16 D: yes
17 - yeah
18 - yeah
→ 19 -- yes there were ten of them
20 S: Gosh
21 D: - *((laughs))*
22 S: so it would have been
23 - pretty intense if you all got together for Christmas *((laughs))*
24 D: oh it was good fun really (.) we
→ 25 -- ah (.) they're you know?
26 they were well spaced out really

(11) Doreen interviewed by Sara, Interview 30 (19 November 2008), (from later in the interview)

	1	D:	mmm,
	2		that's right.
	3	S:	yeah.
»	4		-- one of your friends.
»	5		-- mmm.
⇒	6		--- what about these days?
	7		what do you tend to [do?*
	8	D:	[what* I do? Oh (.) ah (.)
	9		- usually go to one of the family
	10	S:	- mmm hmm
	11	D:	- they take turns or
→	12		-- something like that
	13	S:	- yup
⇒	14		--- oh it's usually a good day
	15	D:	- yes oh yes it's usually a good day
	16		---

The total number of pauses in the first interview with Doreen on 8 February 2007 and in the thirtieth interview on 19 November 2008 is shown in Table 4.4. The second interview is shorter than the first because Doreen was no longer willing to talk for as long as in the early interviews. Because of the different lengths of the interviews, the table also shows the number of pauses per minute for each speaker and overall.

Over the 22 months between the two interviews, the total number of pauses per minute decreased slightly (from 9.7 to 8.4). Although

Table 4.4. Pause length in two interviews with Doreen and Sara, Study 2

	Words turns length	Pauses	*Doreen*: Total pauses	Pauses per minute	Sara: Total pauses	Pauses per minute	Total pauses	Total pauses/ minute
Interview 1	3139	<2 sec	163	6.1	79	0.4	242	6.4
(Feb. 2007)	225	>2 sec	7	0.3	11	3.0	18	0.7
	26:46	Total:	170	6.4	90	3.4	260	9.7
Interview 30	800	<2 sec	65	3.7	55	1.3	120	4.1
(Nov. 2008)	71	>2 sec	7	0.4	23	3.1	30	1.7
	17:46	Total:	72	4.1	78	4.4	150	8.4

Doreen's total number of pauses decreased markedly from 170 in the first interview to 72 in the thirtieth, her number of pauses per minute decreased less dramatically from 6.4 to 4.1. Sara's total number of pauses also decreased between interviews (from 260 to 150), but her number of pauses per minute actually increased in the thirtieth interview (from 3.4 to 4.4). As Doreen's interaction skills decreased, Sara left more time for her to respond. The most striking increase is in Sara's short pauses, which were usually turn internal, as she continued her turns after Doreen did not take up a potential transition relevance place. This can be seen in lines 4 and 5 of Extract (11) (marked by »). Sara leaves two pauses for Doreen to continue her train of thought and then, after a longer pause, moves the topic forward.

There is also a change in the pattern of long pauses. In the first interview, five of the long pauses occurred when Sara fixed the tape recorder or Doreen searched for her diary, leaving a total of 13 long pauses that were within or between utterances. In the thirtieth interview, Sara did not need to fix the tape recorder and Doreen did not look for her diary. All of the 30 long pauses in the thirtieth interview were genuinely within or between utterances: all of Sara's long pauses occurred as she waited to give Doreen adequate time to continue her turn; whereas Doreen's pauses were utterance-internal as she worked out how to carry on. In Extract (11) line 12, after a pause of over one second, Doreen used a general extender ("something like that") when she could not retrieve more content.

A two-second pause is a long time in a conversation, and most people would hurry to fill the silence. It was Sara's training as a speech language pathologist that taught her to allow such long pauses. She also used her knowledge of Doreen's history acquired during her interviews over the 22 months to encourage Doreen to speak more. In Extract (10), when Doreen seems to have stopped talking about Christmases in the past, Sara says "because your husband he came from a large family didn't he?" (line 14). It is noteworthy that Sara gives the information ("your husband he came from a large family") followed by a tag question ("didn't he?") rather than simply asking about Doreen's husband's family directly (see also Karakostas et al. 2010; Davis and Maclagan 2010). This means that Doreen does not have to search for this initial information. After saying "yes" once (line 16) and "yeah" twice (lines 17 and 18), with short pauses, Doreen leaves over a second's pause and adds "yes, there were ten of them" (line 19). Because Sara was able to provide the initial content that the husband came from a large family, Doreen is able to add the extra information that there were in fact ten of them. But she still requires pauses before she is able to retrieve this extra information.

Study 2: Summary

Over 22 months, the language of someone with Alzheimer's disease will usually deteriorate. Unless those who interact with them are skilled, interactions will become considerably less satisfying for both partners. Sara could not prevent the deterioration in Doreen's language ability, but she could ensure that interactions with Doreen continued to last for more than a couple of interchanges. These conversations still occasionally provided information that was new to Sara, but usually they repeated material that Sara already knew and Doreen enjoyed remembering. Although Doreen did not have a memory book, the photograph album allowed Sara to gain important information about Doreen and her family early in the series of interviews, when Doreen could still remember the details. When Doreen's memory became less reliable, Sara knew how to provide the relevant information, or ask a tag question rather than a simple wh-question so that Doreen could continue her turn. Sara's other important skill was her ability to allow longer pauses so that Doreen had time to retrieve the information she could still remember.

Overall Conclusion

As a person's language and memory decline with the progress of Alzheimer's disease, caregivers become increasingly important in holding and retelling the life stories of people with the disease. People with Alzheimer's disease retain their identity and remain more than mere care recipients as long as family members and caregivers know their life stories and help them keep these memories alive. The two studies presented here highlight the importance of the caregiver having information about the life of the person with Alzheimer's disease. In Study 1, memory books were created for Evie, George, and May so that caregivers and others who interacted with them had factual information about their lives as a basis for conversations. Over the relatively short time span of Study 1, the use of memory books allowed Evie, George, and May's conversations to improve.

Such improvements, however, cannot be sustained long term for people with Alzheimer's disease, as seen in Study 2, where Doreen's language decreased markedly over 22 months. In Study 2, information was gained from a family photo album rather than a formal memory book, and this allowed Sara to continue to hold conversations with Doreen, even when Doreen could no longer volunteer the information herself. Successful reminiscing depends not only on the conversational partner's knowledge of the story, but also on the strategies used to keep the conversation flowing. Caregivers should avoid "testing" people with Alzheimer's disease about what they know or remember because this places undue cognitive burdens on them. A deeper knowledge of the person and his or her life story will allow the caregiver to prompt retelling of stories that the person with Alzheimer's disease has shown to be central to his or her identity.

Practical Implications

The two studies presented here show ways in which caregivers can support people with dementia when their life stories must be handed over to others for retelling. A memory book with photos and text that tell the story of the person's life can provide a framework to support continuing interaction with the person with dementia. However, providing a memory book for people with dementia is not sufficient to guarantee improved life story conversations.

Caregivers need specific and individualized training for positive changes to occur. Ideally, such training should be customized for each caregiver, but three relatively simple changes will make a marked difference (see also Dijkstra et al. 2002; Davis and Smith, this volume).

- Leave longer pauses when interacting with older people in general and with people with Alzheimer's disease in particular. Even relatively long pauses are not necessarily indicators of turn completion.
- Avoid asking factual questions about the person's earlier life (*What work did you do?*). Instead, offer information for agreement (*I think you were a typist when you were younger*).
- Avoid asking wh-questions (*Who came to see you this morning?*) which tax the person's already compromised short-term memory. Rather, tag questions (*Your daughter came to see you this morning, didn't she?*) or so-comments (*So, your daughter came to see you this morning*) provide content that helps to stimulate the memory of a person affected by Alzheimer's disease and lets that person respond more easily.

Appendix: Transcription Conventions

(.)	micropause, shorter than 0.5 of a second (brief pauses at the end of utterances are not indicated)
(0.0)	measured pauses or gaps in tenths of seconds
-	indicates a pause less than 1 second long
- -	indicates a pause longer than 1 second but less than 2 seconds
- - -	indicates a pause longer than 2 seconds
< >	brief feedback comments from one speaker inserted during the speech of the other person
~	indicates an incomplete word
?	indicates a question or rising intonation
[	indicates the point at which the utterances that follow are produced in overlap
*	indicates the point at which the current turn emerges from overlap
(xxx)	unintelligible
=	latched utterances without overlap or pause
((laughs))	double parentheses and italic type indicate behaviors or events other than speech that are relevant to the interaction or comments made by the transcriber
Christmas	underlining indicates a marked added emphasis

Notes

We thank the participants in the conversations, without whom the two studies on which this chapter is based would not have been possible. We also thank our research assistant, Sara Blackmore, who carried out and transcribed the interviews for Study 2.

[1] For more details on residential care in New Zealand see: http://www.everybody.co.nz/page-0cf9b494-cf93-4ee1-8db8-aa3b2e527fbd.aspx

[2] See also: http://www.helpguide.org/elder/alzheimers_disease_symptoms_stages.htm

[3] Recordings in the first study were made on a Panasonic DVD video recorder (VDR-D250) with a Panasonic lapel microphone (RPVC200). In the second study they were made on a Sony Minidisk Walkman recorder (MZ-NH1) with a Sony lapel microphone (ECM-C115) and converted to wav files.

References

Andrews-Salvia, M. D., N. Roy & R. M. Cameron. (2003). Evaluating the effects of memory books for individuals with severe dementia. *Journal of Medical Speech: Language Pathology* 11(1). 51–9.

ANZI (Alzheimer's New Zealand Incorporated). (2008). *Dementia Economic Impact Report 2008*. Wellington, New Zealand.

Ash, S., P. Moore, L. Vesely & M. Grossman. (2007). The decline of narrative discourse in Alzheimer's disease. *Brain and Language* 103(1–2). 181–2.

Badkar, J., P. Callister & R. Didham. (2009). *Aging New Zealand: The Growing Reliance on Migrant Caregivers*. Wellington: Victoria University.

Baldwin, C. (2006). Narrative ethics and ethical narratives in dementia. In A. Burns & B. Winblad (eds), *Severe Dementia*, 215–26. Chichester, West Sussex, UK: John Wiley & Sons.

Boersma, P. & D. Weenink. (2009). *Praat: Doing Phonetics by Computer*. Computer analysis program, available from www.fon.hum.uva.nl/praat/. Version 4.6 or later was used for the analysis in this paper.

Bourgeois, M. S. (1990). Enhancing conversation skills in patients with Alzheimer's disease using a prosthetic memory aid. *Journal of Applied Behavior Analysis* 23(1). 29.

—(1993). Effects of memory aids on the dyadic conversations of individuals with dementia. *Journal of Applied Behavior Analysis* 26(1). 77–87.

—(2007). *Memory Books and Other Graphic Cuing Systems: Practical Communication and Memory Aids for Adults with Dementia*. Baltimore: Health Professions Press.

Boyd M., M. Connolly, N. Kerse, S. Foster, M. von Randow, R. Lay-Yee, C. Chelimo, J. Broad, N. Whitehead & S. Walters-Puttick. (2009). *Changes in Aged Care Residents' Characteristics and Dependency in Auckland 1988 to 2008. Findings From OPAL 10/9/8: Older Persons' Ability Level Census*. Auckland: The University of Auckland.

Brooker, D. (2004). What is person-centred care in dementia? *Reviews in Clinical Gerontology* 13(3). 215–22.
Butler, R. N. (1963). The life review: An interpretation of reminiscence in the aged. *Psychiatry* 26. 65–76.
Careerforce. (2008). *Demonstrate Knowledge of Dementia, Person-Centred Care and Communication for a Person Living with Dementia.* Trainee assessment portfolio. 23920 V1, Unit Standard for the National Certificate in Community Support Services (Residential). www.careerforce.org.nz/assets/files/CF%2023920%20V1%20TAP%20no%20bleed.pdf (last accessed 18 September 2010).
Chertkow, H. & D. Bub. (1990). Semantic memory loss in dementia of the Alzheimer's type: What do various measures mean? *Brain and Language* 113. 397–417.
Coleman, P. G. (1999). Creating a life story: The task of reconciliation. *The Gerontologist* 39(2). 133–9.
Crystal, D. & D. Davy. (1969). *Investigating English style.* Bloomington, IN: Indiana University Press.
Davis, B. H. & M. Maclagan. (2009). Examining pauses in Alzheimer's discourse. *American Journal of Alzheimer's Disease and Other Dementias* 24(2). 141–54.
—(2010). *Conversing While Sitting: The Impact of Different Question Types on Conversation.* Paper presented at New Zealand Speech Therapists' Association Conference, Wellington, 22–23 April 2010.
Davis, B. H., M. Spake & T. Gray. (2010). When the picture talks: Creating monogram booklets for spouses and friends. *Activities Directors Quarterly for Alzheimer's Disease* 11(1). 33–38.
Department of Statistics (2009). *QuickStats About Pacific Peoples* www.stats.govt.nz/census/2006censushomepage/quickstats/quickstats-about-a-subject/pacific-peoples.aspx (last accessed 18 September 2010).
—(2010a). *Estimated Resident Population of New Zealand.* Wellington, New Zealand: Department of Statistics. www.stats.govt.nz/methods_and_services/population_clock.aspx (last accessed 24 May 2010).
—(2010b). *National Population Projections: 2009 (base)–2061.* Wellington, New Zealand: Department of Statistics. www.stats.govt.nz/browse_for_stats/population/estimates_and_projections/NationalPopulationProjections_HOTP09base-61.aspx (last accessed 22 March 2010).
Dijkstra, K., M. S. Bourgeois, R. S. Allen & L. D. Burgio. (2004). Conversational coherence: Discourse analysis of older adults with and without dementia. *Journal of Neurolinguistics* 17(4). 263–83.
Dijkstra, K., M. S. Bourgeois, G. Petrie, L. Burgio & R. Allen-Burge. (2002). My recaller is on vacation: Discourse analysis of nursing-home residents with dementia. *Discourse Processes* 33. 53–76.
Fazio, S. & D. B. Mitchell. (2009). Persistence of self in individuals with Alzheimer's disease: Evidence from language and visual recognition. *Dementia* 8(1). 39–59.
Folstein, M. F., S. E. Folstein & P. R. McHugh. (1975). Mini-mental state: A practical method for grading the cognitive state of patients for the clinician. *Journal of Psychiatric Research* 1975(12). 189–98.

Gordon, E., M. A. Maclagan & J. Hay. (2007). The ONZE corpus. In J. C. Beal, K. P. Corrigan and H. Moisl (eds), *Models and Methods in the Handling of Unconventional Digital Corpora: Volume 2, Diachronic Corpora*, 82–104. Basingstoke, Hampshire: Palgrave Macmillan.

Gubrium, J. F. (2005). The social worlds of old age. In M. L. Johnson, V. L. Bengtson, P. G. Coleman & T. B. L. Kirkwood (eds), *The Cambridge Handbook of Age and Aging*, 310–15. Cambridgeshire, U.K.: Cambridge University Press.

Jordan, L., L. Bell & K. Bryan. (2000). *Communicate: Evaluation of a Training Package for Carers of Older People with Communication Impairments.* London: Middlesex University/University College London.

Jorgensen, D., M. Parsons, M. Gundersen Reid, K. Weidenbohm, J. Parsons & S. Jacobs. (2009). The providers' profile of the disability support workforce in New Zealand. *Health and Social Care in the Community* 17(4). 396–405.

Karakostas, T., B. Davis, M. Maclagan & S. Hsiang. (2010). Walking and conversing: Gait and speech adaptations to perturbing direct questions in dementia. *Parkinsonism & Related Disorders* 16(1). S11–86, S49.

Kempler, D., A. Almor, L. K. Tyler, E. S. Andersen & M. C. MacDonald. (1998). Sentence comprehension deficits in Alzheimer's disease: A comparison of off-line vs. on-line sentence processing. *Brain and Language* 64. 297–316.

Kitwood, T. 1997. *Dementia Reconsidered: The Person Comes First.* Maidenhead, Berkshire, UK: Open University Press.

Leichtman, M. D., Q. Wang & D. B. Pillemer. (2003). Cultural variations in interdependence and autobiographical memory: Lessons from Korea, China, India, and the United States. In R. Fivush & C. A. Haden (eds), *Autobiographical Memory and the Construction of a Narrative Self: Developmental and Cultural Perspectives*, 73–98. Mahwah, NJ: Lawrence Erlbaum.

Ministry of Health. (1997). *Guidelines for the Support and Management of People with Dementia.* Wellington, New Zealand: Ministry of Health. www.nzgg.org.nz/guidelines/0045/Guidelines_For_People_With_Dementia.pdf (last accessed 12 February 2009).

—(2002a). *Dementia in New Zealand: Improving Quality in Residential Care.* Wellington: New Zealand Ministry of Health.

—(2002b). *Health of Older People Strategy.* Wellington, New Zealand: Ministry of Health.

—(2004). *Disability support services in New Zealand: The workforce survey.* Wellington, New Zealand: Ministry of Health.

Nicolas, M., L. Obler, M. Albert & N. Helm-Estabrooks. (1986). Empty speech in Alzheimer's disease and fluent aphasia. *Journal of Speech & Hearing Research* 28. 405–10.

Ripich, D., M. Wykle & S. Niles. (1995). Alzheimer's disease caregivers: The FOCUSED program: A communication skills training program helps nursing assistants to give better care to patients with Alzheimer's disease. *Geriatric Nursing* 16(1). 15–19.

Singer, J. A. & P. Blagov. (2004). The integrative function of narrative processing: Autobiographical memory, self-defining memories, and the life story of identity. In D. R. B. J. M. Lampinen (ed.), *The Self and Memory. Studies in Self and Identity*, 117–38. New York: The Psychology Press.

Spilkin, M. L. & D. Bethlehem. (2003). A conversation analysis approach to facilitating communication with memory books. *Advances in Speech-Language Pathology* 5(2). 105–18.

Surr, C. A. (2006). Preservation of self in people with dementia living in residential care: A socio-biographical approach. *Social Science & Medicine* 62(7). 1720–30.

Temple, V., S. Sabat & R. Kroger. (1999). Intact use of politeness in the discourse of Alzheimer's sufferers. *Language and Communication* 19. 163–80.

Ulatowska, H., Allard, L., Donnell, A., Bristow, J., Haynes, S., Flower, A. & A. North. (1988). Discourse performance in subjects with dementia of the Alzheimer type. In H. Whitaker (ed.), *Neuropsychological Studies of Non Focal Brain Damage*, 108–31. New York, NY: Springer-Verlag.

Ulatowska, H. & S. Bond Chapman. (1991). Discourse studies. In R. Lubinski, J. Orange, D. Henderson & N. Stecker (eds), *Dementia and Communication*, 115–32. Philadelphia, PA: B. C. Decker.

Wayne, M. & J. Segal. (2009). *Signs, Symptoms, and Stages of Alzheimer's Disease.* www.helpguide.org/elder/alzheimers_disease_symptoms_stages.htm (last accessed 26 March 2010).

Wilson, J. (2009). Rest home roulette. What are your chances of finding good rest home? *Consumer* 494. 26–9.

Wong, P. T. & L. M. Watt. (1991). What types of reminiscence are associated with successful aging? *Psychology and Aging* 6(2). 272–9.

Chapter 5

From Home to Institution: Roles, Relations, and the Loss of Autonomy in the Care of Old People in Denmark

Trine Heinemann

Introduction

Research on communication in old people's care typically illustrates how, in this context, everyday life is formally administered through institutional routines (Grainger 1990; Gubrium 1975; Lindström and Heinemann 2009; Makoni and Grainger 2002; Somera 1995). Several studies show that old people's care is characterized by an institutional asymmetry between those that give and those that receive care (Ryan et al. 1995), with institutional requirements taking precedence over the individuals' needs and wishes (Backhaus 2009; Heinemann 2009). Such findings are well in line with the observation that the "institution of old people's care" is what Goffman (1961) termed a "total institution": a place where there is a clear split between "staff and inmates," with "inmates" having little or no contact with the outside world, where all aspects of the inmates' lives are conducted in the same place and under the same authority, and where all phases of a day's activity are scheduled.

Goffman (1961: 23), however, also emphasized that human beings are not born into a total institution, but enter as full-fledged members of a "home-world," with a "way of life and a round of activities taken for granted until the point of admission to the institution." Similarly, Nussbaum (1993), with special regard to eldercare, argued that old people go through a transition upon entering a care facility and that the initial interactions that take place between staff and new residents are part of this transition, where the loss of independence about to be experienced by the old person is highlighted.

This chapter, too, explores how old people are socialized into the role of care recipients, but does so by comparing the communicative behavior of old people and their caregivers at the point at which the former have just entered an institution of caretaking, with the communicative behavior of old people who have been part of the same institution for a longer period. Using conversation analysis (see, for instance, Heritage 1984) and focusing on video recorded interactions in the Danish home help system of old people's care, the chapter illustrates how the roles of—and relations between—old people and their caregivers change over time, with an ensuing decrease in the home help receiver's autonomy and an increase in the institutional asymmetry.

The chapter is organized as follows: First, a general introduction to the Danish system of old people's care is given. Then, the difference between "newcomers" and "inmates" is illustrated through an analysis of the communicative behavior of old people and their caregivers in three different situations: (i) the initiation of a visit, (ii) the exchange of food and drink, and (iii) the giving of advice. Having shown that in each of these situations there are significant differences in how the interaction is organized, depending on whether the old person is in an early or late stage of caregiving, and that these differences reflect the change in roles and relations that takes place in caregiving over time, the chapter concludes with a discussion of what consequences this might have for old people and their caregivers, as well as some suggestions for how to address this.

Eldercare in Denmark

With a population of just over five million, Denmark faces the same kind of demographic challenges as other modern societies: 23% of the population is over 60, and with a life expectancy of about 80 and an official retirement age of 65, more than one fifth of the population is on permanent retirement schemes (Danmarks Statistik 2007). People between 65 and 80 receive pensions, social health care and other types of benefits amounting to 192 billion Danish Kroner per year, or more than 10% of the Gross National Product (Danmarks Statistik 2007).

In Denmark, virtually all old people's care is publicly funded and free to the care recipient. About 200,000 old citizens receive some form of care. Old people typically enter the institution of caretaking through the home help system. This system was originally introduced in order to allow people to stay in their own homes as long as possible. It consists of health care workers and social workers, who visit the old people in their own home and assist them with everyday tasks such as cleaning, cooking, and personal hygiene. The typical projection of home-based care is an initial two hours of help per week with practical tasks such as cleaning. Over time, and as the old person's physical and mental abilities decrease, the service is increased to include help with personal care for up to 20 hours per week (Danmarks Statistik 2007).

Because the home help system is based on the belief that autonomous living ensures a better quality of life, admittance to nursing homes is only granted once an old person is deemed to be in danger to him/herself or others, typically when diagnosed with Alzheimer's disease or severe dementia, though this may vary from council to council. As a result of this policy, less than 20% of old people who receive care do so in a nursing home. The typical care recipient in Denmark is thus one who receives some form of help in his/her own home. The existence of the home help system provides a unique opportunity to explore how old people are institutionalized into the care system, because the system encompasses a diverse group, ranging from those that receive what I will here term "early-stage home help" (i.e., people who have just entered the system and receive as little as two hours of help with practical tasks) to those that receive "late-stage home help" (i.e., people who have been in the system for a longer period of time, receive up to 20 hours of help with virtually everything, and are, perhaps, in the process of moving into a nursing home).

In the following, I examine how the interaction between caregivers and early- and late-stage care recipients differs in ways that clearly indicate that old people undergo a socialization process when entering a care institution. I will illustrate this by looking at three different situations: (i) how the visit is initiated; (ii) how food and drink is "exchanged"; and (iii) how the giving of advice is managed. As will be demonstrated in the following, there are systematic differences as to how these activities are managed, depending on whether they occur in early- or late-stage home help. The examples discussed come from a database of video recorded with the participants' consent over a period of half a year and spanning 13 home help visits. These extracts have been chosen for illustrative purposes and can be taken as representative of the database as a whole.

Initiation of the Home Help Visit

The initiation, or opening, of an interaction is the first instance in which participants can define, negotiate, or confirm their respective identities and their interpersonal relations. This has been attested numerous times for telephone conversations (Drew and Chilton 2000; Hopper and Drummond 1992; Schiffrin 1977), but has been argued to be of crucial importance also in face-to-face institutional interactions, such as doctor–patient consultations. Thus, Stivers (2001, 2009) shows that the way a pediatrician initiates the pediatric consultation, for example, is consequential for what role the child will play throughout the rest of the consultation. As will be demonstrated below, roles and relations are also clearly negotiated and defined in the beginning of a home help visit.

As with many other activities performed in home help, entering a care-recipient's home is regulated by institutional guidelines: caregivers should announce their presence by knocking on the door or ringing the bell, and only enter the house upon permission. This procedure not only protects the caregiver from a situation of illegal entry, but also serves to acknowledge that the caregiver is entering the care recipient's *home*, thus preserving some degree of autonomy on the part of the care recipient. In early-stage home help, these institutional guidelines are always respected. By contrast, in late-stage home help, while using the bell or knocking on the door, caregivers may enter the house of the care recipient without waiting for permission. This is illustrated in the following example, where a caregiver rings the doorbell, enters the home of the care recipient, puts her bag on the floor in the entrance hall, starts moving towards the care recipient in the living room and inquires whether the care recipient is hungry—all before the doorbell has stopped ringing. (See the Appendix for the transcription conventions.)

(1) "Ringing the bell" [late-stage care]

1		(*CG rings the doorbell*
2		(*CG enters the hallway and puts down her bag*)
3	CG:	*Ahhh.*
4		(1.3)
5	CG:	*Sulten?*
		Hungry?
6		(0.6)
7	CR:	*Hva' si'r du?*
		What did you say?
8		(0.5)
9	CG:	*Sidder du å' læser salmebog?*
		Are you sitting and reading the hymnbook?
		(*the doorbell stops ringing*)

There may, of course, be very practical reasons why caregivers in late-stage home help do not wait for permission to enter. Care recipients at the late stage are often bedridden or in some other way incapacitated, and hence unable to come to the door and open it. The care recipient in Extract (1), for instance, has severe problems with her legs and is unable to move around without help. Her inability to open the door, however, does not prevent her from being mentally capable of denying or allowing the caregiver entrance to her home.[1] The caregiver could thus choose to enter the hallway but then wait for the care recipient to accept her presence/entrance with a verbal acknowledgement. By entering the door prior to any acknowledgement and in particular by failing to wait for that acknowledgement before entering the living room where the care recipient is sitting, the caregiver ends up using the doorbell not as a request for entering, but as a statement of intent to enter—a unilateral move that need not be ratified by the care recipient. In this way, autonomy is taken away from the care recipient, who in this situation literally has no say in who can enter her house at what time.

The caregiver's unilateral move of entering in late-stage home help not only decreases the care recipient's autonomy, but also raises the issue of what kind of relationship the care recipient and the caregiver have entered into. As mentioned earlier, late-stage care recipients typically receive a significant amount of help, as much as 20 hours a week. As the home help system seeks to ensure that care recipients are visited by as few different caregivers as possible, this means that a care recipient and his/her caregiver typically develop a relationship of familiarity over time and evolve joint routines with which to move through their daily program. That the caregiver in Extract (1) enters without waiting for permission may thus be a reflection of the fact that she is by now so familiar with the care recipient that she can enter in that manner, just as, for instance, the daughter of the care recipient might do. But whereas a unilateral entrance by a daughter or close friend might serve to highlight an intimate relationship, the caregiver's unilateral entrance in late-stage home help also serves to highlight the institutional nature of the visit, in particular when compared with the way in which the same activity is performed in early-stage home help. The subsequent organization of openings in early- and late-stage home help further illustrates this. In late-stage home help, the caregiver typically initiates the first institutional task almost immediately upon entering, as in Extract (1), line 5, where the caregiver inquires whether the care recipient is hungry and then moves towards the kitchen and starts preparing lunch. The caregiver here shows a clear orientation to what she is there for—that is, what her institutional tasks are during this visit. In stark contrast to this, early-stage visits are characterized by a much less restricted organization, in which there is no obvious orientation to the institutional nature of the visit. In the following case, for instance, the caregiver and the care recipient engage in talk about a knitting project that the care recipient wishes to start, immediately after the caregiver has been admitted to the care recipient's home. This explicit move into something that is *not* an institutional task is initiated by the care recipient, who first invites/instructs the caregiver to sit down, then announces that they "should relax for a couple of minutes" (lines 1–3).

(2) "Knitting" [early-stage care]

1 CR: *Sæt- sæt li' døj nå [w.*
Sit- sit down for a [moment.
2 CG: *[Ja,=*
[Yes,=
3 CR: *=.hh Vi ska' li' slappe av to minutter.*
=.hh We'll just relax for a couple of minutes.
4 (0.9) (*CG sits down*)
5 CR: *Å'e:h (1.1) Jæ vi gjerne strikke en bluse te' mig selv.*
Ande:h (1.1) I would like to knit a blouse for myself.
6 CG: *Je [rh.*
Ye[ah.
7 CR: *[.hh Å' det ska' være bomuldsgarn.*
[.hh And it has to be cotton.

Extract (2) shows both care recipient and caregiver orienting to the care recipient's individual needs and wishes as something that is of relevance for the visit. The care recipient here easily overrides any potential institutional requirements and engages the caregiver in small talk. Studies of communication in institutional settings have emphasized the important role such talk plays in allowing the participants to create relations that are not primarily institutionally defined (Toerien and Kitzinger 2007; Backhaus, this volume). In addition, small talk can strengthen the affiliation between participants, help to mitigate or avoid problematic situations (Heinemann 2007), and even serve to elicit information that would not otherwise be available (Burnard 2003). In the context of elderly care specifically, small talk provides a place for the older person to engage in interaction when the inability to leave her home has largely reduced her opportunities for socializing with other people (See Williams (this volume) for an overview on the importance of socializing.).

In Extract (3) the previously discussed small-talk sequence has been completed and the caregiver moves on to initiate the first institutional task. In contrast to how this was done in the late-stage visit of Extract (1), the caregiver here does not simply initiate a task but explicitly inquires of the care recipient what she wants done, thus treating the task as negotiable rather than institutionally predetermined. Once again, the care recipient overrides any institutional requirements by using this opportunity to initiate an entirely non-institutional activity, namely that of drinking coffee.

(3) "What do you want done" [early-stage care]

1	CG:	*Jah, Hva' ve' d* [*u ha'* *laven?*]
		Right, what do [you want done?]
2	CR:	[*Jahmene::h*] *vi ska::* *j'* *ha'*
		[Yes but e: : h] we'll just have a cup
3		*en tår kaffe, =Vi ska' ha'n orn'li' tår kaffe,*
		of coffee you know, = We'll have a proper cup of coffee,

From the very beginning of the home help visits, significant differences are observed in how the roles and relationships of care recipient and caregiver are defined through interaction, depending on whether the visits are done at an early or late stage of the care recipient's progression through the care system. In early-stage home help, the fact that the visit is to the care recipient's *home* is clearly acknowledged by the way in which the caregiver enters and initially engages with the care recipient. By requesting permission to enter (i.e., by knocking or by ringing the doorbell, then waiting for the care recipient to ratify this move), the caregiver clearly takes on the role of a visitor and ascribes autonomy to the care recipient as someone who is entitled to decide who enters her home. By engaging in small talk, rather than initiating the first institutional task, the caregiver similarly refrains from immediately enacting her "institutional role," further treating the visit as a social, rather than primarily an institutional event. This is also reflected by the caregiver leaving it up to the care recipient to decide what they are about to do —for instance, to sit down and have a cup of coffee first as part of "being social."

The caregiver initiating the first institutional task in an open-ended, negotiable manner is also a way of ascribing autonomy to the care recipient, thus casting her in the role of someone who has needs and wishes that may take precedence over institutional requirements. By contrast, in late-stage home help, the fact that the caregiver is an institutional representative whose main purpose is to perform certain institutional tasks is clearly defined, *in particular* by the way in which she immediately initiates the first institutional task, but also through the way in which she enters the care recipient's home. Thus in late-stage home help the care recipient has become to some degree an "inmate" of an institution that once used to be her home.

Exchanging Food and Drink

Another activity in which roles and relations are reflected is the exchange of objects. Such exchanges can in general be done verbally in two ways: either A can offer B an item or B can request an item from A. Studies of interaction have demonstrated that these two ways of exchanging an item are not equal alternatives: offers are preferred over requests (Curl 2006; Schegloff 2007). In the context of old people's care, this asymmetrical relation between requests and offers plays a special role in that it also signifies the relationship between care recipient and caregiver. Previous research has shown that the ability to make requests is crucial to care recipients because it helps to shape their "immediate social environment" (Lindström 2005: 213) and thus constitutes one way in which a care recipient can express her needs and wishes and attempt to have them fulfilled. On the other hand, requests are also one of the activities that serve to highlight the institutional relationship between care recipient and caregiver, inasmuch as the care recipient is entitled to make at least certain categories of requests (Heinemann 2006) by virtue of her institutional role. By contrast, offers—at least those made by the care recipient—typically downplay the institutional context and highlight the fact that care recipients, as inhabitants in their own home, are hosts who can offer certain services or items to the caregiver (Heinemann 2005). The exchange of items thus illustrates different aspects of relationships and roles, depending on which party is doing the offering or the requesting.

In principle, caregivers are not allowed to receive any gifts or services from care recipients. In order to avoid ambiguity, this ban extends even to things like cookies, coffee, and so on. Nevertheless—and as already attested in Extract (3)—care recipients routinely offer food or drink to the caregiver, and such offers are typically accepted. Extract (4) provides another example.

(4) "Piece of rye bread" [early-stage care]

1 CR: *Ve' i hva'¿ ve' i ikk' godt ha' et hajlt*
You know what¿ Won't you please have half a slice
2 *stykke råwbrø?=for jæ' ska'¿=.hhh [Vi ska'*
of rye bread= because I'm having some¿ [We'll
3 CG: *[Jo så*
[Yes then
4 CR: *li' hå't-]*
just have a-]
5 CG: *ta'r vi li' e]t halvt stykke å',*
we'll just take] half a slice as well,

This interaction is from an early-stage home help visit. As can be seen, the care recipient here casts herself in the role of the hostess offering food or drinks. In late-stage home help visits, by contrast, the organization of this exchange is very different. With growing length of regular interaction, food and drink become treated as things that need not be offered, but are there for the taking. This is illustrated in the following two cases. In the first example, something that appears to be an offer of coffee is made by the care recipient. Her turn, however, is formatted very differently from the offers in Extracts (3) and (4). It is in fact formulated as a noticing of an absence (Schegloff 1988) through the use of the modal verb *skal* ("shall," here translated as "are"), which implies that something that ought to be the case has been observed not to apply. Thus, the care recipient is not so much offering coffee as pointing out the caregiver's failure to help herself to coffee. This is also evident in the caregiver's response, which both disconfirms the absence noticed by the care recipient (through the *jo* ["yes"]) and explicitly states that she has helped herself to coffee already. Both care recipient and caregiver in this late-stage visit thus treat coffee as something that need not—indeed ought not—be offered.

(5) "Coffee" [late-stage care]

1 CR: *Ska' du ikk' ha' kaffe?*
Aren't you having coffee?
2 CG: *Jo jeg har taget,*
Yes I've taken some,

Care recipients who are still in their own home pay directly for all items that they need. There should be no confusion, then, about who owns the coffee in Extract (5) and, thus, who has the principled right to administer it. Examples such as this, however, suggest that coffee and other food items—along with the care recipient and her home in general—have been incorporated into the institution to a degree where the boundaries of what belongs to whom are unclear, and where things such as coffee are as accessible to the caregiver as to the care recipient. Thus the exchange of food and drink may in fact have become so routine at this stage that the caregiver can take their availability for granted in the same fashion as we could imagine a close family member could do.

In addition, the physical disabilities of the care recipient in late-stage home help may have an impact on how food and drink is exchanged, inasmuch as the caregiver in these kinds of visits has, in physical terms, better access to food and drink than the care recipient. However, the physical disability of the care recipient does not prevent her from *offering* food or drink (as she indeed at least partially attempts to do in Extract (5)). Neither is the caregiver in any way prevented from asking permission to help herself or to announce that she has done so, thus acknowledging in at least a minimal manner that they are in the care recipient's home and that the food and drink ultimately belongs to the care recipient. The way in which the caregiver in Extract (5) treats the care recipient's noticing suggests that even this possibility for control has disappeared, diminishing the care recipient's ability to act as a hostess. This is further highlighted in the following extract, where a caregiver takes on the role of hostess in the care recipient's home. Here, two caregivers are present and one of them offers the other coffee —an offer that is audible to the care recipient, as is also evidenced from her subsequent comment.

(6) "Yes please" [late-\stage care]

```
1  CG1: Ve' du  ha'  en tår kaffe  Mette?
        Do you want some  coffee Mette?
2       (0.2)
3  CG2: Jah,
        Yes,
5  CR:  Ja  tak     hedder det.
        It's called yes please.
```

In this case then, the caregiver (CG1) does not merely show that she takes for granted her own access to the care recipient's coffee, but she furthermore casts herself in the role of hostess by offering coffee to the other caregiver (CG2). That she does so in the presence of the care recipient in effect means that the latter is denied this role in her own home. Perhaps in an attempt to resist this, the care recipient in this case tries to impose the role of guest on the caregiver who receives the coffee, by correcting her initial ratification of the offer from a simple "yes" to a "yes please" (in line 5).[2]

Despite the general institutional proscription against caregivers receiving anything from care recipients, the exchange of food and drink is something that is taken for granted in both early- and late-stage home help visits. In early-stage home help visits, care recipients' offers of food and drink have an almost routine quality to them and clearly show the care recipient's expectation that their offers will be accepted. As such, the exchange of food and drink, even in these visits, has to a certain degree become institutionalized, inasmuch as such exchanges are part of the (unofficial) agenda for the visit. Despite this institutionalization, however, participants in the early-stage caregiver visits still go through the procedure of producing offers and accepting them. In doing so, they cast themselves and each other in roles that are different from those defined through the institution, namely as host and guest. As such, they manage, at least for a short while, to create a relationship with each other outside the boundaries of the institution. Once a care recipient has moved into the phase of late-stage home help, however, even this minimal reprieve from the institution has disappeared. In late-stage home help, food and drink is thus treated as an integrated part of an institutional whole rather than as something belonging to the care recipient, and as such as something that need not be offered but is there for the taking.

Giving Advice

The third activity in which there is a clear difference between early- and late-stage home help is that of advice-giving, that is, when the caregiver attempts to provide some sort of advice to the care recipient. Previous studies have shown that advice-giving is a sensitive and potentially problematic activity, even in contexts where it is ostensibly the *purpose* of the interaction, for instance in tutor sessions (Waring 2007) or HIV counseling (Silverman 1997). The problematic nature of advice-giving appears to be grounded in the asymmetry that is created between the advice giver and the advice recipient, which ascribes a certain set of competences to the former while implying a lack of competence in the latter (Heritage and Sefi 1992; Hutchby 1995).

Whereas asymmetries in competences and knowledge may be a real factor in meetings between professionals and laymen (Heritage 2008), the kind of competences or knowledge that caregivers have is not specialist knowledge as such. Rather, when caregivers give advice, it is about ordinary everyday things, such as what to eat, how to store food, or how to handle electrical appliances and lit candles. These are all topics that we, as members of a society, would under "normal" circumstances expect other individuals (except perhaps very small children) to know about. Hence, giving advice on these issues is potentially even more problematic than when, for instance, midwives give advice to first-time mothers (Heritage and Sefi 1992).

One way in which to manage the potential problem of giving advice is to package the advice in ambiguity, so that the advice-giving activity is less explicit. This can be done in a variety of ways, for instance through giving accounts for why the advice is given (Waring 2007), or by packaging the advice as something more "innocuous," like providing information. In my sample data, advice from the caregiver to the care recipient is typically initiated in the second way, through the noticing of a "B-event" (Labov et al. 1977). In the following example from an early-stage home help visit, for instance, the caregiver verbally notices that the care recipient has a lit candle in the window of the hall.

(7) "Light in the window" [early-stage care]

1 CG: *>Du ve' godt d'har< lys herover forresten?*
>You do know that you've< got a light here by the way?
2 (0.8)
3 CR: *Ja:h,*

Yes,
4 (0.2)
5 CG: *Nå : h,*
Right,
6 (0.4)
7 CR: *A' jeg har lys hvar?*
That I have got a light what?
8 CG: *Ja i vinduet¿*
Well in the window¿
9 CR: *Jah det har [jeg jo tænd]t* (0.2) *Det har jeg tændt jo,*
Yes that have [I JO lit] (0.2) That have lit JO,
10 CG: [*Nå f'j'ka-*]
[Right because I ca-]

By noticing something verbally, a speaker moves that "something" into the "common ground" (Clark and Schaefer 1989) that he/she shares with the co-participant, so that it becomes available to both and can thus be talked about. "Noticings" can be fairly innocuous activities, employed merely to give the participants in an interaction something to talk about. However, when a speaker notices something that is clearly—and primarily—available to the other, participants will typically look for other reasons why it is introduced (Schegloff 1988). In Extract (7), for instance, there is plenty of evidence for the fact that the care recipient already was aware of the lit candle before the caregiver produced the noticing, and thus that the noticing must have been done for other reasons. First, the caregiver designs the noticing as a stipulation, rather than as an inquiry into what the care recipient knows. In other words, her noticing indicates her belief that the care recipient in fact does know—and does have access to the fact—that there is a lit candle in the window. In turn, the care recipient in her response in line 9 clearly marks this as something she *already* knew, first by stating that she is the one who lit the candle (and hence would know that it is lit), second by including the epistemic adverb "*jo*" in her response, with which she marks the information she provides as already available to the caregiver (Heinemann et al., in press). In the continuation of Extract (7), which is given in Extract (8), and in particular in the care recipient's statement that "she always has a candle there" and "nothing can happen from it," it becomes clear what reason the care recipient finds for the caregiver making the noticing—namely, that she wishes to warn or at least indicate that it might be problematic or dangerous to have lit candles in the window (or perhaps anywhere).

(8) "Light in the window" (continued) [early-stage care]

11	CG:	*(Nå:h)*	
		(Right)	
12	CR:	*Der står lys alti',*	*Der ka' itt' ske no'e' me' det,=*
		There's light there always,	Nothing can happen from it,=
13	CG:	*=Nej det ka' der vel ikk',*	
		=No I guess not,	

Extract (8) is thus an example of how a caregiver, through noticing something that is already available to both herself and the care recipient, can introduce an item with the implicit intention of advising the care recipient on how to deal with this item. It is also clear from Extract (7) that the caregiver treats this kind of action as potentially problematic by the way in which she formulates the noticing. Part of the delicacy with which this advice is delivered may have to do with the *matter* that is advised upon. Noticing that the candle is lit may thus also imply something about the care recipient's (lacking) cognitive abilities, as it indicates that she might have forgotten or that she is incapable of realizing the potential danger of having a lit candle in a window. This is clearly a delicate issue to raise and one that may have significant institutional consequences, as a negative evaluation of a care recipient's cognitive abilities usually results in admission to a nursing home. Whatever the reason, the care recipient here rejects the implicit advice by first claiming her awareness of the light (line 9) and the routine nature of it being lit (line 12), then by stating that this is unproblematic (line 12).

The example in Extracts (7) and (8) is typical of how advice is delivered and received in early-stage home help and, as was the case for the activities discussed in previous sections, the participants' organization of this activity shows an orientation to the fact that the care recipient should be treated as an autonomous person with ordinary competences and rights. By contrast, advice-giving in late-stage home help is typically delivered and dealt with in a manner that does not acknowledge these issues, as Extract (9) illustrates. Here, the caregiver also makes a noticing of something that should be clearly available to the care recipient, namely that the latter has failed to eat her morning snack. In contrast to the previous, early-stage example, however, the caregiver here does nothing to concede to the fact that this knowledge is already available to the care recipient, but designs the noticing as if it were indeed news. In addition, the caregiver immediately turns the noticing into something that is accountable, by inquiring what reasons the care recipient has for failing to eat her snack (line 4), and finally rejects the care recipient's account ("I haven't felt like it") by stating that the care recipient needs to eat (regardless of whether she feels like it or not).

(9) "Morning snack" [late-stage care]

```
 1 CG: Du  har ikk'  gjort  no'et'  ve'  det  mad,
       You haven't done anything about that food,
 2     (0.5)
 3 CR: Nej.  (    [      )]
       No.   (    [      )]
 4 CG:            [Hvor  ]for?=Har    du    sove?
                  [Why?  ]=Have  you  been  sleeping?
 5 CR: Næj.
       No.
 6     (0.4)
 7 CR: Det har jeg  ikk' mæ'  jeg har  ikk'  haft  lyst.
       I  haven't   but   I   haven't  felt  like  it.
 8     (0.7)
 9 CG: Arh  du   ska'   da ha'  lidt  å'  spise  [ Maren¿ ]
       Arh  you should really  eat a little food  [ Maren¿]
10 CR:                                            [Ja: d   ]et  sku'  jeg.
                                                  [Ye: s   ]I   should.
```

In late-stage home help visits, it thus appears that advice-giving is not treated as a problematic activity per se. Instead, advice is delivered in a way that clearly positions the caregiver as the expert with the appropriate competence to say what is, or is not, good for the care recipient, while the care recipient is treated almost as a child who is unable to determine for herself what is necessary. This asymmetry is reflected also in the care recipient's response in line 10, where she accepts the caregiver's advice by agreeing that she ought to eat something.

Discussion

The extracts have illustrated how care recipients and caregivers organize the three activities of openings, the exchange of food and drink, and advice-giving differently, depending on whether the care recipients are receiving home help at an early or late stage in their care history. During early-stage care, the extracts show how visits are initiated in a manner that treat the care recipient as an independent and autonomous person who has the right and ability to decide who enters her home, and as someone who has rights, inclinations, and needs that may take precedence over institutional requirements. Initiations of visits in early-stage home help were furthermore handled in a manner that reflected the fact that the visits take place in the care recipient's *home*, rather than within an institution. Similarly, in the context of exchanging food and drink, it was observed how, in early-stage home help, the participants treat this activity as a social event in which the care recipient can further develop her role as host and the caregiver that of a guest, again with the result that the institutional roles and requirements are downplayed. Finally, the third activity, that of advice-giving, showed how both participants treated this activity as potentially problematic because of the asymmetric relationship it may impose—that is, the caregiver by formulating the advice in a sensitive manner, the care recipient by rejecting the implied advice.

In late-stage home help, by contrast, all three activities were organized very differently. The most noteworthy features identified in the examples discussed are (i) the institutional asymmetry between care recipient and caregiver, (ii) the preference of institutional requirements over individual needs, (iii) a clear and stable definition of institutional roles, and (iv) a lack of ascribed autonomy to the care recipient. This suggests that at this point the care recipient has been almost completely 'institutionalized', despite the fact that she is still living in her own home. The caregiver enters the care recipient's home without waiting for permission to do so, immediately initiates the first institutional task without checking whether the care recipient has other needs or wishes, helps herself (and others) to food and drink, and finally, provides advice in a manner that does not treat the care recipient as someone who has the competence to administer everyday aspects of her life by herself.

Nussbaum (1993: 244) argued that in nursing homes, the institutionalization of the old begins during the admission process, where interactions are organized in a manner that sends "a clear message that a move into a nursing facility is a move into total dependence." The management of the three activities illustrated here further attests that the broad issue of institutional asymmetry, with all that this may encompass, is not *inherent* to old people's care, but is something that is gradually acquired over time through a process that both care recipient and caregiver are engaged in, among other things through their communicative practices.[3]

The question then is whether this process is simply a reflection of a care recipient's deteriorating physical or mental health, or whether the process of institutionalization is also, in part at least, caused by familiarization and the development of joint routines over time. The question, therefore, is whether care recipients in late-stage home help are no longer treated as competent members of society because they *are* no longer competent, or whether activities such as those described above have become so routine—even ritualized—over time that participants in the home help interactions no longer bother to maintain even the most minimal degree of social distance towards each other. This distinction matters. Other studies suggest that helplessness (and thus dependency) is something that can be learned (Rodin and Langer 1980), and that decline in both physical and cognitive abilities can be caused by the loss of autonomy (Aud and Rantz 2005; see also Williams, this volume). In other words, the loss of autonomy that clearly takes place in the home help visits over time could be the *cause* of both physical and mental decline in care recipients, rather than the *result.*

Practical Implications

Loss of autonomy can cause old people in care to become more dependent on their caregivers than is strictly necessary. This may negatively affect their cognitive and social competence. Health care workers thus need to adjust their communicative practices in ways that ascribe the greatest possible degree of autonomy to the receivers of their care. The basic premise of such communicative practices seems to be that old people are competent individuals who, while receiving care help, are *also*, and perhaps primarily, hosts in their own home.

Treating care recipients as independent and competent human beings who are able to take responsibility (at least to a certain degree) for their own lives might have beneficial results over and above "merely" creating a nicer work and living environment for caregiver and care recipient respectively. Ultimately, it may even result in an increase, or at least the retention, of an individual's competence and independence, which in turn may decrease the amount of time and money needed for the caretaking system.

Appendix: Transcription Conventions

The conventions are a modified version of those used by Jefferson (2004).

. , ¿ ?	:	Period, comma, question mark, and inverted question mark indicate, respectively, falling, slightly rising, rising, and strongly rising intonation at the end of an utterance.
(care)	:	Text in parentheses indicates transcriber's uncertainty about what is actually being said or who said it.
[care]	:	Square brackets indicate overlap, that is, places where more than one speaker speaks at the same time.
(1.0)	:	Numbers in parentheses indicate the length of a silence or pause in tenths of a second.
ca::re	:	Colons indicate that a sound or a word is produced in an elongated fashion. The more colons, the greater the elongation.
>care<	:	Arrows indicate that a word or phrase is spoken faster than the normal speed of the speaker.
ca-	:	Hyphens indicate that a word is cut off mid-production.
=	:	Equal signs between words or phrases indicate that there is no gap or beat between the production of the two items.

Notes

I am indebted to Peter Backhaus and Ben Matthews for their extremely insightful and helpful comments on earlier versions of this chapter. I hope I have done these comments justice. Any remaining faults are entirely mine.

[1] Neither does this inability prevent her from using a technological solution, such as an electronic door opener. Such technology has not, however, been installed.

[2] There is no indication in the delivery of this statement that the care recipient intends her reproach to be humorous.

[3] The fact that, in contrast to Nussbaum's study, this study examines caretaking in the context of the old person's own home rather than in a nursing home may further emphasize the gradualness of institutionalization.

References

Aud, M. A. & M. J. Rantz. (2005). Admissions to skilled nursing facilities from assisted living facilities. *Journal of Nursing Care Quality* 20(1). 16–25.

Backhaus, P. (2009). Politeness in institutional elderly care in Japan: A cross-cultural comparison. *Journal of Politeness Research* 5. 54–71.

Burnard, P. (2003). Ordinary chat and therapeutic conversation: Phatic communication and mental health nursing. *Journal of Psychiatric and Mental Health Nursing* 10. 678–82.

Clark, H. H. & E. F. Schaefer. (1989). Contributing to discourse. *Cognitive Science* 13. 259–94.

Curl, T. (2006). Offers of assistance: Constraints on syntactic design. *Journal of Pragmatics* 38. 1257–80.

Danmarks Statistik. (2007). www.dst.dk (last accessed 9 September 2010)

Drew, P. & K. Chilton. (2000). Calling just to keep in touch: Regular and habitualized telephone calls as an environment for *small talk*. In J. Coupland (ed.), *Small Talk*, 137–62. New York: Longman.

Goffman, E. (1961). *Asylums*. New York: Random House.

Grainger, K. (1990). Care and control: Interactional management in nursing the elderly. In R. Clark, N. Fairclough, R. Ivanic, N. McLeod, J. Thomas & P. Meara (eds), *Language and Power*, 147–57. London: Centre for Information and Language Teaching.

Gubrium, J. 1975. *Living and dying at Murray Manor*. New York: St. Martin's Press.

Heinemann, T. (2005). *Requests and Offers: Some Uses of Negative Interrogatives* (MOVIN Movin Arbejdspapirer / Movin Working Papers 2005:3). http://movinarbejdspapirer.asb.dk/pdf/Heinemann2005.pdf (last accessed 9 September 2010).

—(2006). 'Will you or can't you?' Displaying entitlement in interrogative requests. *Journal of Pragmatics* 38(7). 1081–104.

— (2007). Professional self-disclosure: When the home help talks about herself. In C. Kerbrat-Orecchioni & V. Traverso (eds), *Confidence/Dévoilement de Soi Dans L'nteraction*, 325–42. Tübingen: Max Niemeyer Verlag.

—(2009). Managing unavoidable conflicts in caretaking of the elderly: Humor as a mitigating resource. *International Journal of the Sociology of Language* 200. 103–28.

Heinemann, T. A. Lindström & J. Steensig. (In press). Addressing epistemic incongruency in question-answer sequences. In T. Stivers, L. Mondada & J. Steensig (eds), *The Morality of Knowledge in Conversation.* Cambridge: Cambridge University Press.

Heritage, J. (1984). *Garfinkel and Ethnomethodology.* Cambridge/New York: Polity Press.

—(2008). Conversation analysis as social theory. In B. Turner (ed.), *The New Blackwell Companion to Social Theory*, 300–20. Oxford: Blackwell.

Heritage, J. & S. Sefi. (1992). Dilemmas of advice: Aspects of the delivery and reception of advice in interactions between health visitors and first-time mothers. In P. Drew & J. Heritage (eds), *Talk at Work. Interaction in Institutional Settings*, 359–417. Cambridge, MA: Cambridge University Press.

Hopper, R. & K. Drummond. (1992). Accomplishing interpersonal relationship: The telephone openings of strangers and Intimates. *Western Journal of Communication* 56. 185–99.

Hutchby, I. (1995). Aspects of recipient design in expert advice-giving on call-in radio. *Discourse Processes* 19(2). 219–38.

Jefferson, G. (2004). Glossary of transcript symbols with an introduction. In G. Lerner (ed.), *Conversation Analysis: Studies From the First Generation*, 13–31. Amsterdam/Philadelphia: John Benjamins Publishing Company.

Labov, W. & D. Fanshel. (1977). *Therapeutic Discourse: Psychotherapy as Conversation.* New York: Academic Press.

Lindström, A. (2005). Language as social action: A study of how senior citizens request assistance with practical tasks in the Swedish home help service. In A. Hakulinen & M. Selting (eds), *Syntax and Lexis in Conversation: Studies on the use of Linguistic Resources in Talk-in-Interaction*, pp. 209–30. Amsterdam: John Benjamins.

Lindström, A. & T. Heinemann. (2009). Good enough: Low-grade assessments in caregiving situations. *Research on Language and Social Interaction* 42(4). 309–28.

Makoni, S. & K. Grainger. (2002). Comparative gerontolinguistics: Characterizing discourses in caring institutions in South Africa and the United Kingdom. *Journal of Social Issues* 58(4). 805–24.

Nussbaum, J. F. (1993). The communicative impact of institutionalization for the elderly: The admission process. *Journal of Aging Studies* 7(3). 237–46.

Rodin, J. & E. J. Langer. (1980). Aging labels: The decline of control and the fall of self-esteem. *Journal of Social Issues* 36. 12–29.

Ryan, E. B., A. Anas, M. L. L. H. Boich. (1995). Communication predicaments of aging: Patronizing behavior toward older adults. *Journal of Language and Social Psychology* 14(1–2). 144–66.

Schegloff, E. A. (1988). Goffman and the analysis of conversation. In P. Drew & A. Wootton (eds), *Erving Goffman: Exploring the Interaction Order*, 89–135. Cambridge, MA: Polity Press.

—(2007). *Sequence Organization in Interaction. A Primer in Conversation Analysis.* Cambridge: Cambridge University Press.

Schiffrin, D. (1977). Opening encounters. *American Sociological Review* 42(5). 679–91.

Silverman, D. (1997). *Discourses of Counseling: HIV Counseling as Social Interaction.* London: Sage.

Somera, R. D. (1995). *Bordered Aging: Ethnography of Daily Life in a Filipino Home for the Aged.* Manila: De La Salle University Press.

Stivers, T. (2001). Negotiating who presents the problem: Next speaker selection in pediatric encounters. *Journal of Communication* 51(2). 1–31.

—(2009). *The Problem with Three: Opening the Medical Visit in Pediatric Encounters.* Paper presented at the International Meeting on Conversation Analysis & Clinical Encounters, Peninsula Medical School, University of Plymouth, UK, 21–23 July.

Toerien, M. & C. Kitzinger. (2007). Emotional labour in action: navigating multiple involvements in the beauty salon. *Sociology* 41(4). 645–62.

Waring, H. Z. (2007). The multi-functionality of accounts in advice giving. *Journal of Sociolinguistics* 11(3). 367–91.

Chapter 6

Cake or Meat?—A Case Study on Dinner Conversations in a Migrant-in-the-Family Household in Germany

Hilke Engfer

Introduction

Contemporary Germany is one of Europe's fastest aging countries. As far as care for older people is concerned, the buzzword in public and political discussions about the nature and quality of professional care is *Pflegenotstand* ("care crisis"). The national care system is frequently reported to be marked by severe deficits, ranging from lack of modernization of the interplay between public interventions and families (as regulated through the long-term care insurance system) to frequently reported abuses and human rights violations in nursing homes. In order to circumvent these problems, an ever increasing number of older people are being cared for in their own homes by live-in care workers from Poland and other Eastern Europe countries (Neuhaus et al. 2009).

This chapter looks at one such example with special focus on the communicative issues involved in such an arrangement. It starts with a short outline of the demographic environment in Germany, putting the so-called "care crisis" into context. This section will be followed by a short introduction into previous research on migrant live-ins in Germany. The chapter then presents an in-depth analysis of a conversation between a migrant live-in worker and a family member about the eating habits of the Alzheimer's patient cared for. The overall aim is to work out the role of the participants' frames in achieving "common ground." Data analysis will show that potentially conflicting frames have crucial effects on the manner in which care is provided, in particular the task of feeding a person with Alzheimer-related eating disorder.

Demographic Background

With 82 million inhabitants in 2009, Germany has the largest population among all 27 EU member states. This population, however, is marked by an aging society, with death rates continuously exceeding the low birthrate of approximately 1.4 children per mother (Destatis 2010; Lanzieri 2009). The German long-term care insurance system was implemented in 1995. It emphasizes the filial obligation to organize eldercare in order to meet the (financial) challenges of demographic change. Benefits include community-based care, payment to family carers, and payment to nursing homes.

According to the 2006 census, 98% of Germans between 65 and 84 years live in private households, of which one third are single-person households. Merely one fifth (18%) of those who are older than 85 years live in nursing homes (see Hoffmann and Nachtmann 2007: 4). In private households, 1.44 million older people have been reported to be in need of care. These individuals are almost exclusively (92%) cared for by family members, with 28% of the families receiving additional professional help in the form of nursing services (see BMFSFJ 2005: 313).

With regard to the predicted demographic changes, including both population aging and changing family structures, it can be expected that non-familial networks will become increasingly important in the future. Furthermore, it can be anticipated that by 2030 the number of people with "fourth age" diseases (Baltes and Smith 2003), in particular Alzheimer's disease and other forms of dementia, will double (see BMFSFJ 2005: 318). Consequently, the demand for 24-hour care services will increase.

However, professional service providers in Germany are expensive, more expensive than the "do it yourself solution" of migrant-in-the-family care (see Lamura et al. 2008). Accordingly, recent estimates say that approximately 50,000 to 60,000 Polish live-ins assist in German home care today (see BMFSFJ 2005: 316), but the actual number is assumed to be much higher, with the majority of migrants not having registered to work.

The Migrant-in-the-Family Model in Academic and Marketing Discourses

While a number of ground-breaking studies have been dedicated to migrant care workers in the Mediterranean area (Anderson 2000; Bettio et al. 2006; Degiuli 2007; Lamura et al. 2008), in Germany this topic has so far received little attention. Research has predominantly been conducted by sociologists in gender and migration studies looking at changes in informal work and networks (Alt 2003; Irek 1998; Pfau-Effinger 2005), the legal status of evolving new networks in the form of Web-based agencies (Karakayali 2010), the feminization of migration (Koser and Lutz 1998), and the "new maid" as a challenge to gender studies (Lutz 2002, 2007; Odierna 2000). However, no research is available so far on the communicative challenges of the migrant-in-the-family care model in everyday social interaction between the parties concerned, namely the live-in, the cared-for, his or her family members, as well as external care providers.

A look at the marketing discourse by agencies specializing in the provision of migrant-in-the-family care reveals that there are very specific images and definitions of relationships in this increasingly popular home care model. Web-based marketing commonly invokes the stereotypical "Polish warm heart" as a strategy to "commodify love" (see Hochschild 1983). Polish women, as well as Eastern European women in general, are framed as helpers who are able to make up, both physically and emotionally, for absent family members because of their "warm heart," their innate ability to care. Thus, according to the agency *seniorcare24* (quoted in Engfer 2009: 291–294) "[t]he ability to care runs in their blood. They are warm-hearted and loving. They care for the elderly person in the same way a family member would do—24 hours each day. Besides, they are much cheaper than nursing homes."

Methodology

The case study presented in this chapter reflects a typical German migrant-in-the-family home care arrangement consisting of a number of family carers and nursing service employees and a migrant live-in. Data were collected through ethnographic fieldwork. Over a period of six months between December 2007 and October 2008, for approximately four days a week, three hours a day, care interactions were observed involving one Alzheimer's patient (called Wilma), three Polish live-ins, three of Wilma's five children, and seven employees of the local nursing service. Conversations were recorded as audio and transcribed following conversation analytic conventions (see Appendix). Participants did not give their consent to video recordings. However, the author took notes of shifts in body postures and gazes during the interactions.

Wilma was diagnosed with Alzheimer's disease in 2006 when she was 74 years old. After a brief stay at a psychiatric unit, her oldest daughter, Gudrun, hired the Polish nurse Elisabeta through an agency in spring 2007 (all names are pseudonyms). By the time of the study in 2007 and 2008, Wilma exhibited many symptoms of advanced stage Alzheimer's disease, including incontinence, weight loss, wandering, sundowning (a range of "abnormal" behaviors such as wandering or mood swings that occur in the late afternoon or evening), and tremors. All of these symptoms are commonly associated with a rapid decline in cognitive functions (Scarmeas et al. 2007). Wilma also exhibited severe speech disorders as well as noticeable declines in "reasoning" and memory skills.

Describing Wilma in this fashion portrays her as a patient suffering from progressive neuro-degenerative brain disorder—someone whose existence has been stigmatized as "drifting towards the threshold of unbeing" (Kitwood and Bredin 1992: 285). Taking linguistic degradation as a hallmark of dementia, the dementia patient's declining ability to communicate with others about past and present events has led some authors to hypothesize an "internal loss of self in dementia" (Small et al. 1998: 292). According to Cohen and Eisdorfer (1986: 22), "the victim of Alzheimer's disease must eventually come to terms with the complete loss of self."

More recently, a focus on narratives and the discursive properties of communication with dementia patients has identified a number of external influences on the preservation of self or personhood in dementia (Kitwood and Bredin 1992; Sabat and Harré 1992; see also Hamilton as well as Ryan and Schindel Martin, this volume). In contrast to the previously mentioned studies and their focus on the internal, neuropathological and neuropsychological decline, studies such as the one by Kitwood (1990) analyze the role of external, social-psychological factors in maintaining personhood. Acknowledging assumptions that self-identity is constituted by and through social interaction (Coupland et al. 1993; Mead 1934), these studies have shown that the way other people interact with a dementia patient has a significant impact on that individual's sense of identity and well-being.

The present study endorses this latter, interactive approach to Alzheimer's disease. Methodologically it works within the framework of conversation analysis (Sacks et al. 1974) and interactional sociolinguistics (Gumperz 1982). While conversation analysis in this study serves to identify trouble-indicating behavior and repair strategies, interactional sociolinguistics is used for an analysis of the sequential organization of nonverbal cues that provide the means of understanding how participants themselves create the context and make sense of the interaction.

Frames Applied by the Participants to the Home Care Situation

Prior to the observations, selected interviews were recorded to provide insight into how participants frame the home care situation. Asked about her mother, Gudrun, Wilma's oldest daughter and guardian, reported that in 2006, when she was 53 years old, she "had to" admit Wilma into a psychiatric unit. She explained that due to Wilma's increasingly aggressive behavior "we couldn't handle her anymore." Gudrun did not want to talk about this experience, but repeatedly stated that it was "horrible" for both Wilma and Gudrun. Faced with the personality-changing effects of Alzheimer's disease on the one hand, and the dissatisfying care facility they had chosen on the other, this event marks a significant experience and a kind of climax in the course of Wilma's disease. Gudrun realized after a few weeks that she could not leave Wilma in the psychiatric unit. She brought her back home, and soon afterwards Polish nurse Elisabeta moved in. Based on the memory of this experience, Gudrun explained that she learned that at all times her mother had to be treated "in a calm and loving way."

Elisabeta, the Polish live-in involved in the conversation extract below, is a trained nurse and experienced in the care of dementia patients. She worked for 35 years in a Polish hospital prior to retirement. In August 2008, the 57-year-old woman had been working for almost one-and-a-half years in this family. Asked about Wilma, she replied that she is able to bear this kind of work because she is a nurse: "A nurse has to be strong." She then continued explaining her life with Wilma in the early days of her disease when Wilma's husband was still alive. She recalled an afternoon when she and Wilma's husband were sitting at the kitchen table. All of a sudden he started moaning: "Oh, the children never visit us." Elisabeta replied: "Mr. F., your children have just left," and with a laughing voice Elisabeta continued to imitate his reaction: "Really? I am stupid. I must have forgotten." She told me this episode about ten times over the course of the observation, always concluding that she thinks that it is very important that Wilma's children visit her, "so that Wilma does not forget that she is a mother." Elisabeta is a mother herself and treating Wilma as such, while framing the overall live-in situation based on her professional experience, helped her to bond with Wilma in the beginning. Asked about Wilma's children, Elisabeta reported: "The family is good. No problems. However, I am not integrated. Don't get me wrong. I have to care for their mommy. But the moment I decide not to return from Poland, another woman will take over."

An Analysis of Conflicting Frames

The analysis of the following conversation extract focuses on the interaction between Elisabeta (E) and Gudrun (G) while they are feeding Wilma (W) dinner. On Saturdays, Gudrun usually visits them and takes over the task of feeding her mother. Prior to her arrival at around 6 p.m., Elisabeta prepares dinner for Wilma and joins them at the table once Gudrun is there. The analysis concentrates on the trajectories of the conflict between Elisabeta and Gudrun concerning Wilma's eating habits.

(1) (lines 27 to 61)

1	E:	*Ja jetzt Mutti nehmen Tabletten (.) ist ein bisschen* Yes, now mum taking new pills (.) is a little
2	G:	*RUHIGER* (glances at W.) CALMER
3	E:	*Ja, ist ein bisschen ruhiger.* Yes, is a little bit calmer.
4	G:	*Wir haben sie jetzt ja glaub ich vor einem MONAT umgestellt, ne?* (glances at E.) I think we changed her medication a MONTH ago, right?
5	E:	*ABER* <clears throat> *jeden Tag ist andere* BUT <clears throat> every day is different
6	=G:	*anders* different
7	E:	*Zum Beispiel HEUTE* <laughs> *das Essen war schlecht.* For example TODAY <laughs> food was bad.
8	G:	↑ *Ehrlich?* (glances at W.) ↑ Really?
9	E:	*GANZE Zeit laufen laufen.* WHOLE time walking walking.
10	=W:	*xxxxx* *xxxxx*
11	=G:	*Ja (.) ja.* (glances at W.) Yes (.) yes.
12	E:	*Gestern war gut. Aber heute ist schlecht.* Yesterday was good. But today is bad.
13	G:	*Hm* Hm
14	E:	*Isch weiß nischt ob das ist WETTER oder weiß isch weiß nischt.* I don't know if it's the WEATHER or what, I don't know.
15	G:	*Aber das hab ich auch gelesen* (glances at E.) But I've read this too
16	=E:	*FÜR MICH IST GUT WIE LAUFEN. Das ist* FOR ME IS GOOD IF WALKING. That is

17	=G:	*Ja* Yes
18	(.)	*ja, ne?* yes, right?
19	G:	*Ja* Yes
20	E:	(.) *BESSER die Mutti bisschen ESSEN bisschen DENKEN* BETTER mum little EAT little THINK
21	=W:	*xxxxxxxxxxxxxxxx* *xxxxxxxxxxxxxxxx*
22	G:	*Ja* (glances at W.) Yes
23	E:	*Mutti gut essen eh gegessen dann ich bin FROH. Aber so* Mum well eat eh eaten then I'm HAPPY. But like this
24	=G:	*Hm* *Hm* Hm Hm
25		*wie heute das isch bin NICH froh* <laughs> (.) *Zu WENISCH* today I'm NOT happy <laughs> (.) Too LITTLE
26	=G:	*Hm* Hm

The conversation extract starts with a brief exchange about Wilma's medication (lines 1 to 7). Elisabeta states that the new medication positively affects Wilma's behavior (line 1). In the following lines, Gudrun's anticipative statement "CALMER" (line 2), the inclusive "we" and the directive "right?" (line 4), as well as simultaneous speech (line 6), all indicate alignment. Both women agree that Wilma is less restless, but that "every day is different" (line 5). Especially this latter information is an observation that is based on Elisabeta's daily experience of living with Wilma for almost one-and-a-half years. Since Gudrun does not live with her mother and thus lacks knowledge of Wilma's daily eating habits, Elisabeta provides information. The high frequency of disagreement markers (line 5: "But" and <clears her throat>; line 7: "For example" and <laughs>) reflects that she, in contrast to Gudrun, rather than an alignment, perceives a "misunderstanding" here (Pomerantz 1984). This can be explained with regard to the lack of shared background knowledge (see Gumperz 1995).

In lines 8 to 15, Gudrun changes her actions and signals misalignment, too. Her clarification request (line 8: "Really?") precedes her disagreement ("But") and her attempt to take over in line 15. The clarification request "Really?" is an immediate response to Elisabeta's statement "The food was bad" (line 7). Whilst Elisabeta's further explanation in line 9 ("WHOLE time walking walking") indicates that she intended to convey that feeding Wilma was problematic, rather than as a comment on the poor quality of the food, this time Gudrun's attempt to repair the conversation by signaling understanding (as previously performed in line 6) is conspicuously absent. Nevertheless, Gudrun's minimal turn in line 13 ("Hm") seems to signal to Elisabeta that she understands her, because rather than further explaining the connection between the medication and its impact on Wilma's restlessness at lunchtime, Elisabeta gives another possible explanation why Wilma did not eat properly (line 14: "WEATHER"). Here, Gudrun unsuccessfully attempts to take over the turn in line 15, stating that she "read this", probably referring to an article or a book about dementia-related eating disorder. However, Elisabeta overlaps her turn and explains how both she (line 23: "Mum well eat eh fed then I'm HAPPY") and Wilma (line 20: "BETTER mum little EAT little THINK") would benefit from regular eating.

Gudrun's high frequency of backchannel cues between lines 24 and 26 precedes turn taking in line 27. Mirroring Elisabeta, Gudrun starts her narration proclaiming that she will also give an example ("for INSTANCE"). What really follows is an account of Wilma's eating and cooking habits when Gudrun and her siblings were young and her mother healthy.

(2) (lines 27 to 61)

27 G: *Aber das is zum BEISPIEL sie hat*
But for INSTANCE she never liked
28 *früher nie gern gekocht, ne? Zwar für uns Kinder und so aber Mutter war*
to cook, right? Of course, for us children, but mother didn't really like
29 *nicht so für Fleisch und so. Die hat lieber immer Kuchen oder so*
meat and stuff. She always prefers cake and stuff
30 *Süßigkeiten. Wa Mama?*
Sweets. Right mama?
31 W: *Ja, frisch*
Yes, fresh

32 G: *Und ich mein immer DANN SITZT das heute auch noch SO drin*
And I always think that today THIS is still INSIDE her

33 W: *Ja, das is wahr*
Yes, that's true

34 G: *Dann WILL DIE NICHT jeden Mittag essen. Dann isst die SO* (.)
And she DOESN'T WANT to eat lunch every day. She eats like THIS then (.)

35 *NE? So wat GEREGELTES und dann Mittagessen und auch noch mit*
RIGHT? Something STRUCTURED and then lunch and also with

36 *DESSERT und PUDDING und so*
DESSERT and PUDDING and stuff

37 *Also (.) da mein ich dann kommt et wie früher dann auch immer so*
So (.) I think she does what she always used to do (.)

38 *Wa Mama?*
Right Mama?

39 W: *Ja*
Yes

40 G: *PUDDING JA (.) FLEISCH nich. Und das ändert sich nicht* (.)
PUDDING YES (.) MEAT no. And this doesn't change. (.)

41 *Also ich könnte jetzt mit der nach dem Essen wenn se nicht isst, wa*
I could take her now if she doesn't eat, right

42 *sofort nach Café M*
straight away to Café M

43 <laughing voice>: *zwei Stückchen KUCHEN (.) da würd die, NE?* (glances at E.)
two pieces of CAKE (.) she would, RIGHT?

44 E: <laughing voice>: *JA JA*
YES YES

45 G: *Die würd den Kuchen essen, der Kaffee STEHT noch nicht da*
She would eat the cake even if the coffee hasn't ARRIVED yet

46 =E <laughing voice>: *JA JA Aber Kuchen gucken* <laughs>
YES YES Just look at cake

47 G: *Da wär das Stück weg (.) Wa MAMA?* (glances at W.)
Simply disappeared (.) RIGHT MAMA?

48 W: *NEE, wa?*
NO, right?

49 G: <laughs>

50 E: *FLEISCH AUCH. Will muss sein*
MEAT TOO. Wants must be

51 G: *IST DIREKT WEG*
IMMEDIATELY GONE

52 E: *Wenn SCHMECKT ihnen GUT dann ESSEN. Nee wenn NISCH* <laughs>
When TASTES GOOD she EATS. If NOT then DON'T

53 =G: *JA*
Yes
54 G: *Das ist direkt weg, wa MAMA?* (glances at W.)
It's gone immediately, right MAMA?
55 *DANN IS DER KUCHEN WEG <loud> WA Schatz?* (glances at W.)
THEN THE CAKE IS GONE <loud> RIGHT darling?
56 W: *Ja, wat willse haben?*
Yes, what do you want?
57 G: <quiet> *Nix will ich haben* (kisses W.)
I don't want anything
58 W: *Dat kannse weg tun*
You can put this away
59 G: <loud> *Hm Hm ALSO DAS IS IMMER NOCH WIE FRÜHER*
Hm Hm SO THIS IS STILL THE SAME AS BEFORE
60 *Was sie früher gerne gemacht haben oder NICH gerne gemacht haben dat is*
What they liked to do in the past or did NOT like to do that is
61 *NACH WIE VOR. Dat sitzt ganz tief drin*
STILL THE SAME. That is deep down inside

In contrast to Elisabeta, who initially highlights the positive effects of the new medication on Wilma's eating habits—thereby contextualizing these as markers of a disorder caused by Alzheimer's disease—Gudrun interprets Wilma's behavior with regard to the biographical knowledge she has of her mother. Based on this knowledge, she constructs Wilma's behavior as a unique personality trait of hers (line 28: "mother didn't really like"), which she has retained to the present day, according to her daughter (line 29: "She always prefers cake and stuff.").

Contrary to Elisabeta, who identified Wilma's restlessness as her main characteristic (line 9: "WHOLE time walking walking."), Gudrun explains two habits she thinks are distinctive about her mother: First, her mother never liked the structured routine of having lunch every day (line 35: "Something STRUCTURED"); second, she always preferred, and still prefers, cake over a typical lunch that includes meat (line 34: "She eats like THIS then"; line 40: "PUDDING YES (.) MEAT no.").

Of special interest are line 30 and line 38, where Gudrun seeks validation from her mother, and thus seemingly co-constructs Wilma's eating behavior in concert and agreement with her. Whilst Gudrun's posture, facing Wilma, and her gaze between lines 30 and 42 signal her "engagement" (see Goodwin 1981) with her mother, her orientation notably shifts to Elisabeta in line 43. Having established this history of her mother's eating habits, Gudrun initiates a topic change, referring to the situation "now" (line 41), thus reconnecting with Elisabeta's account of Wilma's behavior "today" (line 7). Whereas in lines 5 and 7 Elisabeta signaled disagreement due to the perceived lack of shared background knowledge, her contributions in line 44 ("<laughing voice>: YES YES") and line 46 ("<laughing voice>: YES YES. But watch cake <laughs>") signal that she actively supports achieving a "common ground" (see Clark 1996) through the shared experience of taking Wilma to a café.

In the last two lines (60 and 61), Gudrun states that "What they liked or did NOT like to do that is STILL THE SAME. That is deep down inside." The newly introduced third person plural form clearly indicates that Gudrun no longer refers to her mother. In fact, the use of "they" seems to refer back to line 15 where Gudrun indicates that she does have a certain knowledge about Alzheimer's patients and probably even about Alzheimer-related eating disorders. In contextualizing Wilma's behavior with typical symptoms of the Alzheimer's disease, she thus (ironically) closes the interaction in exactly the same way Elisabeta opened it.

Discussion

The analysis has shown that Gudrun and Elisabeta frame the live-in situation and their relationship to Wilma based on different perspectives: personal experiences and childhood memories in the case of Gudrun, professional experiences and everyday care interaction in the case of Elisabeta. The frames they apply are a result of an ongoing adaptive learning process that is closely linked with the progression of Wilma's disease. In Gudrun's case, her experience of Wilma's stay at a psychiatric unit is engrained in the strategy to treat her mother in a "loving and calm way," which functions as one of her main care strategies. Elisabeta, by contrast, consciously manages interactions with regard to her work experience as a nurse ("I can stand this kind of work because I am a nurse"). By the time Elisabeta moved in, Wilma already exhibited a number of behavioral changes typical of the early stages of Alzheimer's disease. Thus, based on her experience and the changes she has witnessed while living with Wilma, to her Wilma's eating habits are a clear marker of the disease and are, therefore, a "disorder." This is in conflict with Gudrun's care strategy that draws on biographical knowledge of her mother's eating habits.

The way Gudrun frames the home care situation also allows for conclusions to what extent her actions are specific to her own goals. It can be argued that Gudrun prioritizes the preservation of a "shell of normalcy" by "restoring" a past version of Wilma in her interactions with Elisabeta and Wilma. The data presented in this chapter do not provide sufficient proof, but Gudrun's significant change in address from "darling" to "mama" in interactions with Wilma seems to signal a shift—with "mama" being more likely to respond to normal/healthy behavior (compare lines 30, 38, 47, 54), and "darling" more likely to occur with trouble-indicating behavior (line 55, preceded by Gudrun's suddenly increased volume in response to Wilma's trouble-indicating silence). In her interactions with Elisabeta, Gudrun indicates twice that she is aware of standardized dementia care practices (line 15: "But I've read this too"; lines 60–61: "What they liked or did NOT like to do that is STILL THE SAME."). However, she contextualizes this information with regard to achieving her overall aim of restoring Wilma's "normal" eating behavior.

Essentially, the analysis of the conversation shows that the distribution of knowledge between the two main carers, Gudrun and Elisabeta, is uneven. Elisabeta's apparent lack of biographical knowledge about Wilma, on one hand, and Gudrun's ignorance concerning the day-to-day business of living with her, on the other, provoke a relationship mismatch between the two carers that affects negotiations of changes for the better within the home care arrangement. As seen in lines 41 to 55, the shared experience of taking Wilma to Café M serves to temporarily create common ground between the two women. That such common ground is considered important by the two interlocutors is testified by Gudrun's subsequent concession to Elisabeta's point of view (line 51), where she acknowledges that Wilma likes meat, too. However, Gudrun's concluding remark about Wilma's unaltered personality traits clearly signals that she is adamant about her original point of view. This shows that the two women are not equal partners who discuss Wilma's eating habits, but hold different positions in the "home care hierarchy," with Gudrun, as Wilma's daughter and Elisabeta's employer, being the head.

Practical Implications

In the care of Wilma, Gudrun and her siblings prioritize comfort and life quality in their mother's care, but a certain amount of "blindness to the facts" makes them the ones who potentially prevent changes that may improve Wilma's quality of life. Gudrun is focused on who Wilma once "was" and rejects certain crucial changes that her disease entails. Being the one who lives with Wilma, Elisabeta's opinions and views are therefore essential. However, the process of communicating, negotiating, and prioritizing interpretations of Wilma's behavior in order to assure the best possible care is potentially problematic.

In the advanced stages of Alzheimer's disease and other dementias, qualified care workers who know how to treat common symptoms are usually part of a home care network. In Wilma's case, Elisabeta reported her eating habits and consequential loss of weight to the nursing service employees who assist her twice a day. External nursing employees thus can function as mediators between migrant live-ins and the family members. A structured way of distributing knowledge between all the individuals involved in a home care system will help assess more appropriately the quality of life and needs of the person cared for. In the present case, this would help the live-in and the family members alike to understand and accept the Wilma who "was" and the Wilma who "is". Family members therefore should provide the live-ins with sufficient biographical information about the care recipient and essential information concerning the progression of the disease, just as live-ins should keep the family informed on a regular basis about their everyday life with the patient.

Contrary to the discourse perpetuated by the employment agencies, migrant live-ins do not simply "replace" absent family members. They fill a crucial gap in the provision of in-home eldercare. However, they rely on assistance and the organized distribution of knowledge in order to achieve—as part of a network—the best possible environment for the person in need of care.

Appendix: Transcription Conventions

<word>	comment on articulation
=	simultaneous talk, when more than one person is speaking at a time
(word)	body posture, activity, nonverbal communication
(.)	micro pause, less than one second long
wo: rd	lengthening of a syllable
x	inaudible syllables
↑	rising tone
WOrd	stressed articulation

References

Alt, J. (2003). *Leben in der Schattenwelt: Problemkomplex "Illegale" Migration.* Karlsruhe: von Loeper Literaturverlag.

Anderson, B. (2000). *Doing the Dirty Work? The Global Politics of Domestic Labour.* London and New York: Zed Books.

Baltes, P. B. & J. Smith. (2003). New frontiers in the future of aging: From successful aging of the young old to the dilemmas of the fourth age. *Gerontology* 49. 123–35.

Bettio, F., A. Simonazzi & P. Villa. (2006). Change in care regimes and female migration: The 'care drain' in the Mediterranean. *Journal of European Social Policy* 16(3). 271–85.

BMFSFJ (Bundesministerium für Familie, Senioren, Frauen und Jugend). (2005). *Alter und Gesellschaft. Fünfter Bericht zur Lage der älteren Generation in Deutschland.* Berlin: BMFSFJ.

Clark, H. (1996). *Using language.* Cambridge: Cambridge University Press.

Cohen, D. & C. Eisdorfer. (1986). *The Loss of Self.* New York: W. W. Norton and Company.

Coupland, N., J. F. Nussbaum & A. Grossman. (1993). Introduction: Discourse, selfhood, and the lifespan. In N. Coupland & J. F. Nussbaum (eds), *Discourse and Lifespan Identity,* x–xxvii. Newbury Park, California: Sage.

Degiuli, F. (2007). A Job with no boundaries. Home eldercare work in Italy. *European Journal of Women's Studies* 14. 193–207.

Destatis (Statistisches Bundesamt Deutschland). (2010). *Durchschnittliche Kinderzahl 2008 in den Neuen Ländern Angestiegen* (Pressemitteilung Nr.034 vom 27.01.2010). www.destatis.de/jetspeed/portal/cms/Sites/destatis/

Internet/DE/Presse/pm/2010/01/PD10__034__12641,templateId=rende rPrint.psml (last accessed on 20 June 2010).

Engfer, H. (2009). Polnische Betreuerinnen in der häuslichen Altenpflege in Deutschland—eine interdiskursive Perspektive. In I. Röskau-Rydel, P. Fischer, B. Kerski, K. Ruchniewicz, M. Krzoska (eds), *Inter Finitimos—Jahrbuch zur deutsch-polnischen Beziehungsgeschichte* 6. 291–4. Osnabrück: Fibre Verlag.

Goodwin, C. (1981). *Conversational Organization: Interaction Between Speakers and Hearers.* New York: Academic Press.

Gumperz, J. (1982). *Discourse Strategies.* Cambridge, MA: Cambridge University Press.

—. (1995). Mutual inferencing in conversation. In I. Markovà, C. F. Graumann & K. Foppa (eds), *Mutualities in Dialogue.* 101–23. Cambridge, MA: Cambridge University Press.

Hochschild, A. R. (1983). *The Managed Heart: The Commercialization of Human Feeling.* Berkeley, CA: University of California Press.

Hoffmann, E. & J. Nachtmann. (2007). *Alter und Pflege. GeroStat Report Altersdaten 03/2007.* Berlin: Deutsches Zentrum für Altersfragen.

Irek, M. (1998). *Der Schmugglerzug. Warschau-Berlin-Warschau. Materialien Einer Feldforschung.* Berlin: Schiller Verlag.

Karakayali, J. (2010). *Transnational Haushalten: Biographische Interviews mit "Care Workers" aus Osteuropa.* Wiesbaden: VS Verlag.

Kitwood, T. (1990). The dialectics of dementia: With particular reference to Alzheimer's disease. *Ageing and Society* 10. 177–96.

Kitwood, T. & K. Bredin. (1992). Towards a theory of dementia care: Personhood and well-being. *Ageing and Society* 12. 269–87.

Koser, K. & H. Lutz (eds). (1998). *The New Migration in Europe: Social Constructions and Social Realities.* London: MacMillan.

Lamura, G., H. Döhner & C. Kofahl (eds). (2008). *Family Carers of Older People in Europe—A Six-Country Comparative Study.* Berlin: LIT Verlag.

Lanzieri, G. (2009). Population and social conditions (*eurostat Statistics in focus* 81/ 2008). http://epp.eurostat.ec.europa.eu/cache/ITY_OFFPUB/KS-SF-08–081/EN/KS-SF-08–081-EN.PDF (last accessed on 27 September 2010).

Lutz, H. (2002). In fremden Diensten. Die neue Dienstmädchenfrage in Europa als Herausforderung für die Migrations- und Geschlechterforschung. In K. Gottschall & B. Pfau-Effinger (eds), *Zukunft der Arbeit und Geschlecht* 61–182. Opladen: Leske und Budrich.

—. (2007). *Vom Weltmarkt in den Privathaushalt: Die Neuen Dienstmädchen im Zeitalter der Globalisierung.* Opladen: Leske und Budrich.

Mead, G. H. (1934). *Mind, Self, and Society.* Chicago, IL: Chicago University Press.

Neuhaus, A., M. Isfort & F. Weidner. (2009). *Situation und Bedarfe von Familien mit Mittel- und Osteuropäischen Haushaltshilfen.* Köln: Deutsches Institut für angewandte Pflegeforschung e.V.

Odierna, (S. 2000). *Die Heimliche Rückkehr der Dienstmädchen.* Opladen: Leske und Budrich.

Pfau-Effinger, B. (2005). Welfare state policies and care arrangements. *European Societies* 7(2). 321–47.

Pomerantz, A. (1984). Agreeing and disagreeing with assessment: Some features of preferred/dispreferred turn shapes. In J. M. Atkinson & J. Heritage (eds), *Structure of Social Action: Studies in Conversation Analysis*, 57–101. Cambridge, MA: Cambridge University Press.

Sabat, S. R. & R. Harré. (1992). The construction and deconstruction of self in Alzheimer's disease. *Ageing and Society* 1. 443–61.

Sacks, H., Schegloff, E. A., & Jefferson, G. (1974). A simplest systematics for the organization of turn-taking for conversation. *Language* 50. 696–735.

Scarmeas, N., J. Brandt, D. Blacker, M. Albert, G. Hadjigeorgiou, B. Dubois, D. Devanand, L. Honig & Y. Stern. (2007). Disruptive behaviour as a predictor in Alzheimer disease. *Archives in Neurology* 64(12). 1749–54.

Small, J. A., K. Geldart, G. Gutman & M. A. Clarke Scott. (1998). The discourse of self in dementia. *Ageing and Society* 18. 291–316.

Chapter 7

"Me Nurse, You Resident": Institutional Role-Play in a Japanese Caring Facility

Peter Backhaus

Introduction

Japan's population is among the oldest worldwide. The ratio of people aged 65 and over tripled from 7.1% in 1970 to 21.5% in 2007. Though Japan's elderly are generally known for their good health, the country's rapid aging in recent years has entailed an ever-growing number of people in need of care. According to the latest figures by the Japanese Ministry of Health, Labour and Welfare (2009), 4.7 million persons are eligible for benefits from the national care insurance. This is no less than 3.7% of the country's total population. More than 826,000 of the entitled persons receive benefits for institutional care services, such as home care, day care, and various sorts of residential care.

Though institutional elderly care is becoming an ever more important issue, little is known as yet about life inside the caring facilities. This holds particularly true for the linguistic properties of institutional care, which only very recently have started to be included on Japanese researchers' agendas (Katō et al. 2004; Kitamoto 2006; Komatsu et al. 2005; Onoda 2007; Suzuki 2001).

This chapter adds to this developing strand of research by taking a closer look at the role relationships between residents and staff as they are played out in interaction between the two groups. Data were collected in a Japanese elderly care facility referred to by the pseudonym "Edogawa Care." Located in Saitama Prefecture on the northern outskirts of the Tokyo metropolitan region, Edogawa Care is officially designated as a "geriatric health care facility" (*kaigo rōjin hoken shisetsu*), one of several types of Japanese caring institutions.

Geriatric health care facilities offer short-stay programs, usually between 3 and 6 months, with a special focus on rehabilitation.

Borrowing from previous approaches to the topic (Gibb 1990; Grainger 1993a; Sachweh 2000; Wadensten 2005), conversations between residents and staff were recorded during the morning care activities. Actions performed during morning care include waking the residents, washing and dressing them, and helping them go to the toilet. The sample consists of 107 mostly dyadic resident-staff conversations recorded by a small digital recorder that was placed in the pocket of one of the care workers on shift. All recordings were made on the second floor of Edogawa Care, which accommodates relatively healthy residents with few or no symptoms of dementia.

The chapter starts with a look at what previous researchers into communication in elderly care have observed with respect to the characteristic features of talk between residents and staff. As will be shown, two basic types of talk can be distinguished by the degree of their groundedness in the institutional context. The main part of the paper discusses two longer extracts of talk from the data recorded in Edogawa Care. The focus is on the different types of role relationships that are constructed and negotiated during the interactions. The concluding discussion summarizes the main findings and derives a few practical suggestions for communication in institutional elderly care, in Japan as elsewhere.

Previous Research

Previous researchers of communication in nursing, both in general and with special regard to elderly care, have developed various taxonomies for the different communicative styles they found in their respective research environments. In many cases these are closely linked to the content matter or topic of a conversation. For instance, Macleod-Clark in her (1982) dissertation on nurse-patient verbal interaction in English hospitals has identified the following content categories: emotional/psychological, treatment/care, intake/output, and social "chit-chat." In quantitative terms she found that over 80% of her sample data were about either treatment/care or intake/

output, and thus directly related to a given caring task (Macleod-Clark 1982: 183).

Bottorff and Morse in a (1994) paper about research on verbal and nonverbal behaviors of nurses during interactions with cancer patients in U.S. hospitals distinguish between four types of attending: (i) "doing tasks," where the focus of attention is exclusively on the task at hand; (ii) "doing with," where the focus is equally on the task and on the patient; (iii) "doing for," where the main focus is on the patient; and (iv) "doing more," where the main emphasis is on the patient's personhood. Bottorff and Morse's terminology was also applied by Wadensten (2005) in a study on nurse-resident communication in a Swedish eldercare facility.

In her dissertation on the rehabilitation of elderly patients in an English hospital, Fairhurst (1981) makes a basic distinction between a "talk to" and a "talk with" mode in nurse-patient interaction. The former includes what Fairhurst calls "ceremonial talk," which aims to "ensure the smooth execution of tasks," as well as "marvelling talk," characterized by excessive praise and encouragement of the elderly patients. The "talk with" mode is observable in what Fairhurst refers to as "time-out talk." It is non-task-related and in her data was mainly reserved for conversations taking place after a given care activity had been completed (Fairhurst 1981: 348–350; similar Fairhurst 1978).

Both verbal and nonverbal interaction was studied by Wagnild and Manning (1985) in geriatric long-term care facilities in Texas. They distinguish between procedural and non-procedural modes of resident-staff interactions during bathing. They studied a total of 42 interactions and found that no less than half of them contained only procedural conversations, or no conversation at all.

The object of analysis in Gibb's (1990) and Gibb and O'Brien's (1990) research on communication in an Australian nursing home was the speech act. Working with audio data collected during morning care activities, a total of 42 types of speech acts used by the nurses were identified. Most frequent were confirmations, explanations, instructions, comments, and inquiries (referred to as "checking out" by the authors). Of special note is the comment category, which differs from the other categories in being a "predominantly social category in which information was shared which had little purposeful intent in terms of getting the job done" (Gibb and O'Brien 1990: 1401). According to Gibb and O'Brien, the fact that comments in the data frequently occur interspersed with other kinds of speech acts

> facilitates a fluid movement between different roles for the resident: on the one hand, as a fairly passive recipient of care, taking directives or accepting explanations about what is being done to them and, on the other, as a participant in a mutual conversational exchange on equal standing with the nurse. (Gibb and O'Brien 1990: 1397)

One of the earliest discourse analytical approaches to communication in institutional elderly care is Grainger's (1993a, 1993b) study of resident-staff interaction in the geriatric wards of two English hospitals. She focused mainly on conversations during getting up and bathing routines, for which she distinguishes four modes of discourse: (i) routine management discourse, (ii) nurturing discourse, (iii) sick/dependent discourse, and (iv) personal discourse. The last differs from the former three in that it is principally noninstitutional and based on solidarity. Thus it allows the participants to "background their institutionally prescribed roles of 'nurse' and 'patient' and to acknowledge each other as individuals" (Grainger 1993b: 254). Personal discourse is commonly marked in Grainger's data by topic shifts to noninstitutional matters such as holiday activities, leisure time, etc.

Among the most recent approaches to the topic is a study by Ward and his colleagues (2008) about interactions in five British care facilities. The authors distinguish between task-based encounters, characterized by a focus on the task at hand, social or relationship-oriented encounters, which were not observably motivated by a pending task, as well as combinations of the two. Their quantitative analysis revealed that 77% of all analyzed encounters were task based, while only 15% were genuinely social or relationship oriented. As the authors observe, "both residents and carers had a tightly-defined role to play in these encounters from which they rarely departed" (Ward et al. 2008: 639).

Though the different taxonomies discussed here reflect different methodological backgrounds and research interests, all of them contain a basic distinction with regard to the participants' role relationships as social actors in an institutional environment. While most of the identified types of talk reflect the participants' roles as caregivers and care recipients, previous researchers also have distinguished types of talk in which the interlocutors temporarily choose to redefine their role relationship on the basis of noninstitutional categories. These two types of talk are summarized in Table 7.1.

The distinction between the two types of talk is not as clear-cut as it is presented here, though. One basic problem arises from the fact that nursing necessarily contains elements of "care" that may be motivated both institutionally (care as service provision) and personally (care as an affective state of mind) (see Makoni and Grainger 2002: 807 for a discussion). For reasons of simplicity, the categorization in Table 7.1 considers merely the former notion of care. As a result, categories such as MacLeod's (1982) "emotional/psychological"

Table 7.1 Institutional vs. noninstitutional role relationships in previous research

Previous research	Institutional role relationship	vs.	Noninstitutional role relationship
Fairhurst (1981, 1978)	• Ceremonial talk • Marveling talk		• Time-out talk
Macleod-Clark (1982)	• Emotional/psychological • Treatment/care • Intake/output		• Social "chit-chat"
Wagnild and Manning (1985)	• Procedural conversation		• Non-procedural conversation
Gibb (1990)	• Confirmation • Explanation • Instruction • Checking out		• Comment
Grainger (1993a, 1993b)	• Routine management discourse • Nurturing discourse • Sick/dependent discourse		• Personal discourse
Bottorff and Morse (1994)	• "Doing tasks" • "Doing with" • "Doing for"		• "Doing more"
Ward et al. (2008)	• "Task-based encounters"		• "Social encounters"

discourse and Grainger's (1993a) "nurturing discourse" have been subsumed as being institutionally motivated even though they may contain elements that go beyond mere service provision.

This relates to a complementary problem. As Grainger (1993a, 1993b) has emphasized, even the occurrence of noninstitutional talk—or, in Grainger's own terms, personal discourse—may be motivated on the part of the staff by a desire to facilitate the care routines. This questions the very existence of a noninstitutional category as such. All in all, however, the distinction between institutional and noninstitutional role relationships is sufficiently straightforward to serve as a vantage point for a closer analysis of linguistic interaction in Edogawa Care. The following will discuss two extracts from the sample in which both types of role relationships can be observed. Special focus is on the shifts between the two during the interactions.

No Need to Keep Quiet

The first example is from a conversation between a female care worker aged 31 and a 79-year-old male resident. The extract[1] starts during the diaper change, with the resident explaining to the care worker why he hasn't called her via nurse call. Despite some splitting pain in his stomach, he says, he decided to wait for her to come by herself.

(1) No need to keep quiet (#82)

1	Res.:	=*aa nandaga, kirikiri hara itai* [###
		I somehow got the gripes (###)
2	Staff:	[*a ieba yokatta no ni,*
		[You should have told me,
3		*yobeba yokat* [*ta no ni*
		you should [have called.
4	Res.:	[*iroiro ne* [*:*
		[Well, I h [ad my reasons.
5	Staff:	[*nande yo:,* (1.9)
		[Why?
6		*(son)na gaman suru koto nai ja nai,* (0.8)
		There is no need to keep quiet.

7 Res.: *iyaiya, itsumo gaman shite ###*
But I'm always keeping quiet (###)
8 Staff: *nandeyo: gaman shinai de yo:*
What are you saying?! Don't do that!
9 (1.4)
10 Staff: *guai waruku nattara komaru kara*
Because if you get sick we'll be in trouble.

In line 1, the resident first mentions the pain in his stomach. The care worker's first reaction on hearing this is to tell the resident that he should have made a call. The resident replies that he had "his reasons" for not calling, upon which the care worker in lines 5 and 6 protests by telling him that there is no need to keep quiet. The original term she uses is *gaman,* which literally means something like "tolerance" or "endurance." It is a frequently used term in Japanese everyday conversations, and is also referred to in the next two lines: First the resident counters the care worker's reproach by telling her that he always keeps quiet. The care worker's reaction is another note of protest ("What are you saying?!") and an unmitigated request in line 8 to the resident to stop doing so.

The most interesting turn occurs in the last line, where the care worker qualifies her previous statement by giving the resident the reasons why she does not want him to keep quiet: Because when he gets sick, they will be in trouble. Due to the omitted subject for the verb *komaru* ("be in trouble," "have a problem"), it is not entirely clear who the nurse thinks would be in trouble in the case of the resident getting sick. It could be the resident, who would no doubt have a problem if he got sick, but it could also be the nurse herself, whose institutional duty it is to take care of the resident's health. A third possible reference could be to the institution as a whole. In order to convey a similar kind of vagueness in the English gloss, the plural pronoun "we" was chosen, which here can be understood as both inclusive ("you and me") and exclusive ("me and the other nurses").

This final statement by the nurse serves to clarify the motives for her kindness and consideration towards the resident and his (unspoken and outspoken) needs. It is not, or not in the first place at least, because she likes him as a person, but rather because she fulfills an institutionally defined role that makes her responsible for him: She is the carer; he is the cared-for. This is not to say that the care worker would not "care" for the resident on a personal level, too, but as her final statement shows, she finds it important to disambiguate the two types of care by invoking her institutional responsibilities. The fact that she delivers this final statement only after a pause of 1.4 seconds (line 9) suggests that there is a certain degree of hesitation about the redefinition of her "caring" relationship with the resident solely on the basis of institutional necessities. Structurally the pause functions as a boundary that marks a shift back from the noninstitutional to the institutional world.

Hot and Cold

The second example features the same care worker, this time in conversation with a female resident aged 75, whose speech shows clear traces of the Kansai dialect spoken in western Japan. The care worker has just entered the room to do the morning care. While opening the curtains she jokingly exchanges the greeting *ohayoo gozaimasu* ("Good morning") with the resident several times, each time with a different intonation. This creates a warm and relaxed atmosphere right from the start.

(2) Hot and cold (#37)

1 Staff: ((Staff enters room and jokingly exchanges greetings
with resident several times while opening the curtains))
oHAyoo gozaima [*su*
Good morning.
2 Res.: [*arama,*
[Oh dear,
3 *kuchi ippai, kao ippai* [*yana* ((laughs))
mouth covered, face covered
4 Staff: [((laughs))
5 *kazeppoi kara ne,*
It's because it feels like I'm getting a cold,
6 *minna ni utsushicha ikenai kara sa* (0.7)
and I don't want to transmit it to everyone.
7 Res.: *kusuri nonderu no?*
Are you taking medicine?

8 Staff: *soo, kusuri nonderu no.*
Yes, I do.
9 Res.: *nonderuno ee kedo,*
Medicine is okay,
10 *anta ue nanka kina:: [sai*
but put some clothes on!
11 Staff: *[atsukutte:*
[It's hot!
12 Res.: *honma nan?*
Really?
13 Staff: *ugoiteru to ne*
When you're moving around.
14 Res.: *naa ase kaku no mo=*
And sweating is also
15 *=waruiya [ne* *[un, sore wa*
bad, isn't it? [Yeah, that's
16 Staff: *[unsoonano* *[yone, de sotoni=*
[Yes, that ['s true, and
17 *=gomi sute ikuto samukut [te*
when I go out to throw away the garbage, it's cold,
18 Res.: *[samukute ne=*
[Cold, isn't it
19 Staff: *=demo sooiu toki ue dake haotteru kara, [chanto*
but I put on my jacket then, so, well
20 Res.: *[sokka=*
[I see.
21 Staff: *=unn=*
Yeah
22 Res.: *=daijoobu?=*
Okay?
23 Staff: *=daijoobu ari [gatoo*
Okay, thank [you
24 Res.: *[un*
[Yeah
25 (1.9)
((sound of wheelchair footrests being opened))
26 Res.: *kaze hiitara naoran ne,*
When you catch a cold you won't get rid of it
27 *kono goro no ## [#nnnakana [ka ne:*
these days [after all [, you know
28 Staff: *[ne::* *[doo shimashoo,=*
[Yeah. [What shall we do?

29		*=okimasuka?*
		Are you getting up?
30	Res.:	*unn, soo, nanji?*
		Yeah, right, what time is it?
31	Staff:	*rokuji mawatta kedo*
		Just turned six.
32	Res.:	*a, hona okiyoo.*
		Oh, let's get up then.

After the joking sequence at the opening the resident moves the conversation on by commenting on the gauze mask the care worker is wearing. Starting with *arama,* translated as "Oh dear" in line 2, the resident almost literally awards her utterance a tone of endearment. The care worker replies to the resident's comment by explaining that she feels like she is getting a cold and does not want to transmit it to everyone (lines 5 and 6). Next the resident asks the care worker if she is taking medicine, which she confirms.

The following turn by the resident (line 10) deserves special attention. While acknowledging that it is important to take medicine, she strongly advises the care worker to "put some clothes on!" Her utterance *anta ue nanka kina::sai* is an imperative, both in form and in function. Added by the term of address she uses towards the care worker, *anta,* a term that is normally restricted to family or other intimate relationships, the resident's way of speaking here much more resembles a mother telling off her daughter than a resident in a care facility speaking to a nurse.[2]

Some degree of self-consciousness about whether this way of speaking is appropriate to the situation can be seen in the resident's lengthening of the verb form *kina::sai.* The resident here obviously hesitates whether or not to produce an imperative, but because the *na* syllable on which she has got stuck is morphologically already part of the imperative form, it is difficult to make something other than an imperative out of this.

As for the care worker, she seems to eagerly take up her part in the assumed mother–daughter play by designing her reply in an almost child-like complaint style: she feels hot because she's moving around all the time (line13), but on the other hand gets cold when having to go out to throw away the garbage (line 17). She even reports that she puts on a jacket on these latter occasions (line 19). Her use of the term *chanto* in this turn, which means something like "properly" or "as one should," further adds to the impression of a child obediently reporting to her mother. The skilful backchanneling behavior by the resident (lines 14–15 and 18) adds to the family-like atmosphere in this part of the conversation.

The mother–daughter sequence continues through another three lines (22–24), in which the resident asks the care worker if she is all right. The care worker replies that this is the case and then thanks the resident for her sympathy, upon which the resident adds a closing token, *un*. This formally terminates the sequence about the care worker's coming cold, and would make this point a good opportunity for a topic shift to the task at hand: getting the resident out of bed. Indeed, as the background noise on the recording suggests (the sound of wheelchair footrests being opened can be heard), the care worker has already started making preparations in this respect.

However, instead of the conversation taking this course, the resident, after a pause of 1.9 seconds, adds a follow-up on the previous sequence by telling the care worker that if she gets sick now, it will be hard to recover. The care worker in line 28 reacts with an emphatically pronounced backchannel token, *ne::* ("Yeah"), and then, while the resident is still speaking, performs a harsh topic shift by asking "What shall we do? Are you getting up?" (line 28). Doing so, she signals to the resident that she is unwilling to continue the personal discourse any further, and wants to concentrate now on the caring task. Her introduction of the new, task-related topic is also marked by a formal speech style (*shimashoo, okimasu*), in contrast to the previous conversation, which was conducted entirely in nonformal style. The topic shift here thus co-occurs with a speech level shift.

The somewhat abrupt way with which the care worker introduces the new topic can best be explained as a result of her growing impatience after the resident's follow-up on the previous topic, which is surplus both in terms of structure (sequence organization) and content (a mere reprise of the resident's motherly concerns). The resident's reaction shows that she immediately understands the care worker's discontent. Her "Yeah" in line 30 is not an answer to the question "Are you getting up?", but a mere token of approval of the just-performed role and topic shift. This becomes clear from the resident's subsequent inquiry ("what time is it?") in the same line, which would not make much sense if asked after having already gotten up. The resident's real compliance "let's get up then" is given only after the care worker has answered her question about the time in line 32. With both interactants talking about the task of getting up now, the shift from personal to institutional discourse has been completed.

Discussion

The two examples show how caregiver and care recipient in and through their linguistic interaction can shift between their institutional and noninstitutional roles. In Extract 1, the resident presents his refraining from using the nurse call as an act of personal benevolence. He knows that the care worker is busy at this time of day and wants to make things easy for her by putting his own preferences last. This degree of considerateness, and particularly the fact that the resident is not particularly eager to conceal it, clearly goes beyond what would commonly be expectable for interlocutors whose relationship with one another is defined primarily on the basis of their institutional roles. The care worker eventually feels the need to remind the resident that the main reason she wants him to use the nurse call is her institutional responsibility rather than her personal preference. This sets the discourse back on the institutional track.

The second example has similar characteristics. The longer mother–daughter sequence right after the opening greeting clearly deviates from common institutional procedures. Usually it is the resident's state of health that is inquired about. Here, however, it is the other way round: The resident asks the care worker about her gauze mask, and the latter willingly and in much detail makes a self-disclosure (see Heinemann 2007) about her coming cold. Both participants are thus actively involved in temporarily redefining their relationship beyond their institutionally assigned roles as carer and cared-for. In the end it is again the care worker who breaks the spell by reminding the resident of the caring task that needs to be performed. Her question *doo shimashoo?* ("What shall we do?") in line 28 functions as a soft but determined push of what could be called the "me-resident-you-nurse" button.

Both cases thus include a temporary suspension or even reversal of the institutional roles ascribed to the two parties. For a moment, the carer becomes the one who is cared for, and the cared-for the one who cares. This produces a greater degree of instability with regard to the interactants' definition and presentation of their role relationship. The same instability is discernible in the small print of the two interactions, both of which contain what could be called "insecurity cues" with regard to the roles chosen, or about to be chosen, by the participants.

In the first example, the care worker's emphasis of her institutional responsibility at the end of the extract ("If you get sick we'll be in trouble") is preceded by a longer pause that suggests hesitation about the statement that is in the making here. Extract 2 contains two similar insecurity cues. The first one is the resident's hesitation about the appropriateness of the imperative ("Put some clothes on"), which she formulates during the mother–daughter sequence. The lengthening of the second syllable of the verb (*kina::sai*) neatly captures her wavering over to what extent she may act out her mother role towards the care worker. The second insecurity cue is the pause after the provisional termination of the sequence. It is obvious here that the two participants construe these almost two seconds of silence very differently. While for the care worker they mark the end of the noninstitutional talk sequence, the resident considers them merely an intermission after which to continue the mother–daughter conversation just a little longer.

Both interactors thus have at their disposal different roles between which they can shift back and forth during the conversation. As a matter of fact, they first and foremost talk to each other as care worker and care recipient, each with a relatively narrowly defined set of expectable verbal and nonverbal behaviors. However, the interlocutors in the course of the interaction look for ways to deviate from these roles and define their relationship in different, noninstitutional terms. Important for these role shifts to happen is that both sides contribute to making them work. As Gibb and O'Brien (1990: 1390) observe in their study in an Australian nursing home:

> The nursing home culture is not prescribed but dynamically constructed and maintained by face to face interaction, chiefly between nurses and residents. Each person shapes the other's behaviour, including communicative behaviour, as they co-operate to achieve certain objectives as part of the activities of daily living for residents in a nursing home.

Practical Implications

Occasional shifts from institutional to noninstitutional talk can fulfill an important function in that they give participants a break from their predefined roles: the nurse from being nurse, the resident from being resident. This reference to a noninstitutional reality can be expected to have positive effects on the mental well-being of both actors involved. Particularly with regard to the elderly person, it may help break up the downward spiral described in the Communication Predicament of Aging Model (Hummert et al. 2004; see also Williams, this volume).

To what extent it is practicable—or recommendable, at least—to talk the caring institution "out of being," as the participants in the two examples try to do, is a difficult question. Though it is no doubt desirable that the relationship between residents and staff should go beyond a mere performance of caring tasks, it cannot be denied that these tasks make up an overwhelming part of the care work as a whole. This will necessarily shape the communication between caregivers and care recipients. What would appear important is to find the right balance between the usual "me-nurse-you-resident" talk and other types of talk that go beyond the interlocutors' institutional functioning.

Notes

I would like to thank Yoshiko Matsumoto and Yuko Sugita for their most helpful comments on earlier versions of this paper. Special thanks to Eileen Fairhurst for kindly finding me a copy of her (1978) paper.

[1] The transcription conventions are largely based on Jefferson (see Atkinson and Heritage 1984: ix–xvi).

[2] As mentioned before, the resident speaks some form of Kansai dialect, which is known to be much more direct than the Japanese spoken in and around Tokyo (e.g., Onoe 2010).

References

Atkinson, John M. & John Heritage (eds). (1984). *Structures of Social Action: Studies in Conversation Analysis.* Cambridge: Cambridge University Press.

Bottorff, Joan L. & Janice M. Morse. (1994). Identifying types of attending: Patterns of nurses work. *Journal of Nursing Scholarship* 26. 53–60.

Fairhurst, Eileen. (1978). *Talk and the Elderly in Institutions.* Paper presented at the Annual Conference of the British Society of Social and Behavioural Gerontology, Edinburgh, U.K., 14–16 September.

—(1981). A sociological study of the rehabilitation of the elderly in an urban hospital. Unpublished doctoral dissertation, University of Leeds.

Gibb, Heather. (1990). 'This is what we have to do—are you okay?' Nurses' speech with elderly nursing home residents (Research Monograph Series 1). Geelong: Deakin University.

Gibb, Heather & Bart O'Brien. (1990). Jokes and reassurance are not enough: Ways in which nurses relate through conversation with elderly clients. *Journal of Advanced Nursing* 15. 1389–401.

Grainger, Karen. (1993a). The discourse of elderly care. Unpublished dissertation thesis, University of Wales.

—(1993b). 'That's a lovely bath, dear': Reality construction in the discourse of elderly care. *Journal of Aging Studies* 7(3). 247–62.

Heinemann, Trine. (2007). Professional self-disclosure: When the home help talks about herself. In Catherine Kerbrat-Orecchioni & Veronique Traverso (eds), *Confidence/Dévoilement de Soi Dans L'interaction,* 325–42. Tübingen: Max Niemeyer.

Hummert, Mary Lee, Teri A. Garstka, Ellen B. Ryan & Jaye L. Bonnesen. (2004). The role of stereotypes in interpersonal communication. In Jon F. Nussbaum & Justine Coupland (eds), *Handbook of Communication and Aging Research,* 2nd edn, 91–114. Mahwah, NJ and London: Laurence Erlbaum Associates.

Katō, Shinji, Tetsuya Abe, Tomoyuki Yabuki, Yoshihisa Abe & Norikazu Nagashima. (2004). Shōkibo kea ni okeru kōkateki kainyū moderu no sakusei [Developing an effective intervention model for small-size care]. In Kōreisha Chihō Kaigo Kenkyū Kenshū Sendai Sentā (ed.), *Chihōsei Kōreisha Oyobi Kaigo Kazoku no Seikatsu no Shitsu no Kōjō ni Kansuru Kenkyū Jigyō* [Research on the improvement of life quality for demented elderly and their families], 117–70. Sendai: Kōreisha Chihō Kaigo Kenkyū Kenshū Sendai Sentā.

Kitamoto, Keiko. (2006). Sōsharu wāku ni okeru komyunikēshon bunseki: Tokubetsu yōgo rōjin hōmu ni okeru seikatsu bamen o chūshin ni [An analysis of social work communication: On daily life conversation at a nursing care home for senior citizens]. *Bulletin of the Graduate School of Josai International University* 9. 49–64.

Komatsu, Mitsuyo, Yasuhiro Kuroki & Yasuko Okayama. (2005). Jūdo ninchishō kōreisha ni taisuru kaigo sutaffu no koekake no tokuchō to koekake puran no kanōsei o saguru [Voice characteristics of speech used by nursing staff and the potential for use in the formulation of care plans]. *Ninchishō Kea Gakkaishi* 4(1). 32–9.

Macleod-Clark, Jill. (1982). *Nurse-Patient Verbal Interaction: An Analysis of Conversations in Selected Surgical Wards.* Unpublished doctoral thesis, University of London.

Makoni, Sinfree & Karen Grainger. (2002). Comparative gerontolinguistics: Characterizing discourses in caring institutions in South Africa and the United Kingdom. *Journal of Social Issues* 58(4). 805–24.

Ministry of Health, Labour and Welfare. (2009). *Kaigo Hoken Jigyō Jōkyō Hōkoku no Gaiyō (Heisei 21-nen 6-Gatsu Zanteiban)* [Provisional report on care insurance services, June 2009]. www.mhlw.go.jp/topics/kaigo/osirase/jigyo/m09/dl/0906a.pdf (last accessed 14 September 2010).

Onoda, Takao. (2007). Kōreisha to herupā no kaiwa no tokuchō ni tsuite [On the properties of conversations between older adults and home helpers]. *Tokoha Gakuen Tanki Daigaku Kenkyū Kiyō* 38. 21–40.

Onoe, Keisuke. (2010). *Osaka Kotobagaku* [Osaka linguistics]. Tokyo: Iwanami.

Sachweh, Svenja. 2000. *Schätzle Hinsitze! "Kommunikation in der Altenpflege."* Frankfurt: Peter Lang.

Suzuki, Seiko. (2001). Kaigo fukushishoku no komyunikēshon sukiru ni kansuru kentō: Jiko hyōka kara [Study on communication skills of care workers through self-estimations]. *Kaigo Fukushigaku* 8(1). 71–8.

Wadensten, Barbro. (2005). The content of morning time conversations between nursing home staff and residents. *International Journal of Older People Nursing/Journal of Clinical Nursing* 14(8b). 84–9.

Wagnild, Gail & Roger Manning. (1985). Convey respect during bathing procedures. *Journal of Gerontological Nursing* 11(12). 6–10.

Ward, Richard, Antony A. Vass, Neeru Aggarwal, Cydonie Garfield & Beau Cybyk. (2008). A different story: Exploring patterns of communication in residential dementia care. *Aging and Society* 28. 629–51.

Chapter 8

Reframing to Regain Identity with Humor: What Conversations with Friends Suggest for Communication in Elderly Care

Yoshiko Matsumoto

Introduction

This chapter looks at how older adults in their verbal interactions with friends and peers depict and deal with various aspects of the transitions they experience at their stage of life, and considers the implications for communication in elderly care. The analysis of casual conversations of older Japanese women with their friends shows that such verbal interactions allow for potentially discouraging experiences of life changes to be recast in a different light, and to be shared with humor and laughter among the participants of the interactions. Such findings are worthy of attention when considering communication in the care offered to older adults. The discourse strategies in the analyzed conversations reveal multilayered and flexible identities maintained and presented by older individuals rather than an identity solely attributable to advanced age or to the role of a care recipient. While much of the data examined is from verbal interactions among individuals who are in relatively good health and thus able to live independently, similar observations can be made in care facilities in the conversations between (healthier) residents.[1] The analysis of such conversations offers insights that are relevant to the provision of care, because the situation of the healthy and independent elderly presents the starting point of a continuous process in which giving and receiving care becomes increasingly relevant.

In the following sections, I will first discuss the findings from casual conversations between relatively healthy Japanese women (aged in their seventies and early eighties) who live independently, with a particular focus on conversations about the topics of illness and death. Contrary to what may be expected from the discouraging nature of such topics, as well as from the gloomy stereotypes associated with the older adult's communication (for a detailed discussion of such stereotypes see, e.g., Coupland, Coupland and Giles (1991)) what is remarkable in the conversations that I analyzed is that these interactions are frequently accompanied by humor and laughter (see also Matsumoto 2005, 2008, 2009). The humor and laughter are produced and sustained collaboratively by the speakers and the hearers, a fact that is in stark contrast to the findings by Jefferson (1984) who claimed that listeners of "troubles talk" do not normally reciprocate the speaker's laughter unless the contents are pleasantries.

Furthermore, the data I examine also reveal that, although there was no humorous comment or laughter when a simple statement about illness or death was first made by a speaker in a conversation, humor and laughter were observed later when the topics of illness or death were taken up again and elaborated on by including memories and descriptions of specific mundane events in that person's life. These findings illustrate that, through focusing on everyday aspects of a "painful" event and thereby reframing the narrative of such an event within a *quotidian frame*, older speakers can present painful life events from the perspective of the mundane matters that they can laugh about and thus eventually alleviate and come to terms with their pain (Matsumoto 2009; forthcoming). This suggests that the disclosure of age-related personal matters does not necessarily carry negative connotations, especially among friends and peers, but instead provides opportunities for the interlocutors to share experiences and enjoy conversations. Reframing "painful" life changes within a quotidian perspective appears to be a means of regaining a sense of the "normal" and "ordinary" self that the interlocutors are familiar with. Such reclaiming of one's "normal" self is likely to be particularly important to those who are undergoing constant transitions in old age. I found similar discourse strategies in the casual conversation of residents of a care facility. This suggests that opportunities for casual and varied conversation are important for older persons to maintain their sense of self and their multilayered identities.

Casual Conversations with Friends and Peers

The observations in this chapter of verbal interactions among relatively healthy older adults are based on audio recordings of approximately 33 hours of casual conversations of four Japanese women (aged in their seventies and early eighties) over a span of 5 years. The conversations involved either a friend or peer aged 65 or older, or a younger friend (i.e., the researcher). The occasions for the peer conversations were not specifically arranged for the purpose of the research but were prearranged independently by the participants as gatherings of friends or volunteer work. One-on-one conversations with the researcher were conducted without a set of planned questions, and the older individuals (who had known the researcher at least over a year and a half) took the initiative in the selection of the topics during the course of the conversations.[2] "Natural" conversations of independent older adults with friends (from the peer group and the younger generation) were specifically collected for the investigation to complement the more controlled verbal data of first-time older acquaintances (Coupland, Coupland and Giles 1991) and of a number of studies on communication with care recipients (Hamilton 1994; Ryan, Hummert and Boich 1995; Davis 2005).

Reframing Conversational Narratives

The main speaker in Extract (1) is Akiko.[3] She was 75 years old at the time of the recording and had lost her husband 7 months prior to this conversation. During the 90-minute conversation, she talked to a younger friend, the researcher, about various topics, including memories of her childhood, her daughter's family, volunteer work, her favorite books, and dramas. In the course of the conversation, Akiko recounts the last moment of her husband's life in two different ways: first in a solemn "key" (in Goffman's term), and later in a humorous key by reframing the narrative as a quotidian event, a presentation that involved laughter.

The very first mention of her husband's recent death occurred as a side remark to Akiko's explanation about how she started watching a popular TV drama. Akiko returned to this topic a little later in the conversation, where she expanded on her husband's passing by retelling various "sub-events" that had occurred in the days leading up to his death, including his long-term health issues, his interactions with the doctor and nurses, and his unwillingness to undergo dialysis. These events she recounted all with a solemn tone of voice which continued for about 60 minutes into the 90-minute conversation to the beginning of the scene in Extract (1), in which Akiko's tone of voice suddenly changes.

The conversation extract starts with Akiko mentioning that her husband passed away quietly in his sleep in a hospital room while she and his doctor were watching a monitor tracking his heartbeat. The mimetic adverbial expression *pu:tto* in line A6, a word that indicates the manner in which something disappears quietly, marks the end of the "story" about her husband's passing away.

Immediately following this, Akiko retells her experience of the same moment again in lines A7 to A16, this time in a tone of animated everyday talk with laughter. She says that, unlike how death scenes are usually depicted in TV dramas, neither did her husband say sweet words nor was there a clear sign of the exact moment of his death. Instead, she says, his last word was telling her to "shush" since he was trying to sleep.

The change of tone in Akiko's recounting is apparent from the use of various linguistic devices which reflect and are used to create interactional involvement among conversation participants (Tannen 1989). For example, in line A7, the repetition of the pragmatic particle *ne* (as underlined in the extract) is used to engage the listener in the talk. In contrast to earlier narratives including the one ending with line A6, in this segment the scene of her husband's death is told in more detail, including "constructed dialogue" (in Tannen's term) or "reported speech." Also in contrast to the previous segment (and the summary of the experience given after line A17), this narrative is delivered in the present (rather than the past) tense, which further increases the involvement of the speaker and the vividness of the description. The content and the chosen linguistic devices together give the impression that Akiko's narrative in this segment is in the form of a regular everyday complaint about her husband's misbehavior, complaints of the general type that wives may tell to their friends in a casual conversation. It may thus be said that the moment of her husband's passing, described in a somber key in all earlier parts of this conversation, is reframed here as a quotidian description: a casual complaint about her husband's usual misbehavior, something that can be told with laughter.

In the extract given below, the instances where reframing can be detected are indicated by a line break. Akiko's utterances are transcribed in the A lines, and those that were accompanied by laughter are indicated in small capitals bracketed with "$". Laughter is indicated with "H" in "< >" and light laughter (or aspiration) is marked by "h". The researcher's responses are transcribed in the Y lines. The temporal positions of back-channeling and laughs indicated in the English translation are approximations necessitated by word order differences between Japanese and English. "###" indicates speech that was indecipherable.

(1) The last moment of Akiko's husband

A1: moo sensei to hutari de saigo mitottan desu yo.

A2: ano, detekudasai mo nan no zya [nai
Y2:   [nakute

A3:   [moo, ano, koo, ano sindenzu no yo[o, monitaa minaga[ra
Y3: ee [ee   [ee ee   [ee

A4: sensei to hutari to kokono ne, ano sizu: kani nemutta mama de [su yo
Y4:   [aa soode

A5: itaku mo kayuku mo nai.

A6: puu: [tto
Y6:   [puu

------------------------- (reframing) -------------------------

A7: sooide atasi ga nee nanka o yuu to ne saisyo no uti ne

A8: netenda kara urusai yo tte [yu < h h >
Y8:   [< H H H H>

A9: urusai koto yuu na toka   ne. sore gurai de
Y9: <   H   H   H   h h   >   ee ee

A10: soo yutte kara atasi ni dakara ariga$TOO TOKA NAN NIMO YU$

A11: urusai kara damattero tte yuu
Y11: < h h h   H h > damattero < h h >

A12: sore ga saigo $NO KOTOBA DATTA TO OMOU KEDO NE$, [honto yo
Y12: [< h h h >

A13: soide ne, neteta no

A14: [un, [yuu
Y14: sore de neru yooni tteyu [u no wa hontoni nanka son [na kanzi

(*Lines omitted*)

A15: de yoku, gaku toka nanka yo [ku terebi a:nna no mo nai no
Y15: [ee: arimasita yo koyuhuuni ne, un

A16: na::ni [are (*in dumbfounded voice*) $DAKARA ATASI$
Y16: [< H h h >

--------- ------------------ (reframing) --------- ----------------

A17: hon: ttoni sensei to hutari de soyatte mite [ta no
Y17: [soo::

A18: daka atasi honttoni, rinzyuu o mitotat [te yu koto aru desyo?
Y18: [ee ee ee ee

A19: hazimeteno keiken desita [ne
Y19: [ee ee

Translation

A1: So, I was beside him with the doctor, watching him at his last moment.

A2: I wasn't asked to go out of the room, [or anything like that
Y2: [You weren't

A3: [So, um, this, um, like ECG, [we were looking at the moni[tor
Y3: uh [huh [uh huh [uh huh

A4: with the doctor, from here, um (my husband) was just quietly sleeping, [y'know
Y4: [oh, I see

A5: there was no pain, no nothing.
A6: wafted [away
Y6: [wafted

--------- ------------------ (reframing) --------- ----------------

A7: and, y'know, when I say something, y'know, early on

A8: "I am sleeping, you are noisy", [he says < h h >
Y8: [< H H H H>

A9: like "don't be noisy" or something like that, y'know
Y9: < H H H h h > uhuh

A10: after all these words, $$HE (DID/DOES)N'T SAY A WORD OF "THANK YOU" TO ME$

A11: "don't be noisy and shush up", he says
Y11: < h h h H h > shush up < h h >

A12: I $THINK THAT WAS HIS LAST WORD$, [really
Y12: [< h h h >

A13: then, he was sleeping

A14: [yes [they do
Y14: passing away as if he fell asleep, [just like people say, [it really felt like that

(*Lines omitted*)

A15: and that motion of the head when someone dies, [which you often see on TV, there isn't anything like that either
Y15: [Oh yes, I know what you mean, like this, right.
A16: what is [tha: t? (*in dumbfounded voice*) SO, I
Y16: [< H h h >

---------- ------------------- (reframing) --------- -------------------

A17: really, together with the doctor, I was watching him [that way
Y17: [I see

A18: so I really, people talk about the [last moment, you know?
Y18: [uh huh uh huh

A19: For me this was the first time I experienced that [you know.
Y19: [uh huh

Throughout the middle part (lines A7 to Y16) of the extract, both the narrator and the hearer laugh without reserve. The laughter seems natural here even though it would not be usually expected that a recently widowed woman talking about her husband's death and the hearer of her narrative would laugh (see, e.g., Jefferson 1984). There are several reasons why this scene is humorous. According to the "incongruity theory" of humor that I pointed out in (Matsumoto 2009; forthcoming),[4] it is both the mismatch between the grave subject matter and the light manner of its presentation that contribute to the humor in the narrative, as well as the incongruity between the regular expectations that people have about the last moment of one's husband's life and the reality of how that death actually happens. In other words, the narrative is amusing in part because the presentation focuses on the perceived ordinariness of the moment of death.

After this humorous part (lines A7 to Y16), the tone of the conversation returns to being somber again in the last few lines (A17 to A19), where Akiko gives a summary by saying that it was the first time for her to closely experience the moment of someone's death. Thus, Extract (1) reveals two changes in the way in which verbal interaction is framed (see, e.g., Bateson 2000 [1972]; Goffman 1974; Tannen 1979), namely from a serious life-changing event to that of a minor quotidian event that can induce and allow for laughter (Matsumoto 2009; forthcoming), and back again to serious narrative. This sort of shifting or "reframing" in conversational narratives (especially reframing into what I refer to as the "quotidian frame") when recounting a psychologically intense experience invokes a feeling of everyday life that can make the atmosphere less tense and give rise to laughter.

Quotidian reframing of a narrated event can be conducted collaboratively, that is, co-constructed among participants of a conversation. This is shown in Extracts (2) and (3), which are from a tea-time conversation among four women in their seventies who share a hobby and, in the two extracts given below, talk about events related to the serious lung condition, including asthma attacks, that the husband of one of the participants, called Tamako, suffered from. Tamako herself introduced this serious topic early in the conversation and in a relatively somber tone without laughter, just as Akiko did in the example above. Later Tamako began to present more details, recounting that her husband played around with the equipment which he was given by his doctor to measure the amount of oxygen as if it were a toy. This narrative of his childish behavior of trying out the equipment on anyone who visited him is a clear instance of quotidian reframing that included constructed speech (reported speech) and laughter.

The collaborative signaling of quotidian reframing by the other participants is noticeable in their various trivial questions about the equipment. For example, when one of the participants called Kimiko asked how oxygen measurement was taken, Tamako replied that she did not know how to operate the equipment, thus causing all participants to burst out laughing.

After a few similar turns, in Extract (2), Kimiko teases Tamako by wondering out loud whether "his wife" had not been helping him in measuring the oxygen count, thus insinuating that Tamako had not been up to the standard of a good wife. The topic is still the serious illness of Tamako's husband, but Kimiko (K) reframes it as a scene about wifely duty in the daily life of a traditional couple and, thus, makes everyone laugh.

(2) Does "his wife" help?

K1: okusama wa zenzen o-tetudai-$SITE NAI NO [KASIRA NE$ <H [H> sono toki ne
H1: [<H H H>
R2: [<H H>

Translation

K1: His wife doesn't help him at all? $I [WONDER $ <H [H> at that time
H1: [<H H H>
R2: [<H H>

Continuing the topic of her husband's life-threatening asthma attacks and the oxygen measurement equipment, Tamako (T) then mentioned a medical procedure that had to be administered within 3 minutes of the occurrence of a particular symptom to save her husband's life. In response to one of the participants' comment that ambulances (usually) do not arrive in 3 minutes (in line H2), a comment that marks the beginning of Extract (3), Tamako, maintaining the quotidian framing, explains how the ambulance always arrived on time, pointing out the obvious fact that her husband would not have been alive otherwise. She reconstructs the ambulance crew's words: "We know well where your house is," implying that they had often been called to Tamako's house, as if they were a delivery service. Tamako describes animatedly that, on these frequent emergency occasions, she would take down the sliding doors so that the stretcher with her husband could be carried quickly into the ambulance. In spite of the serious life or death situation, everyone's tone is noticeably jocular as indicated by the amount of laughter.

(3) Arrival of ambulance
T1: so.
K1: sonomama ni sitoku to moo, anoyo ittyau wake?
H2: nee, sositara san pun inai ni kyuukyuusya konai zya nai.
T3: demone $DAI [TAI$, < h >, $MAIKAI KITERU KARA IKITERU NO$.

K3: [< H H H H H H >
R3: [< H H H H H H H >

T4: [su,
H4: [kiteru no?
R4: < H H H H H H >

T5: eee? <H H H H h h > moo, o,
H5: < H H H H H H H H H H H>
K5: < H H H H H H >
R5: iya iya < H H H H H HH HH>

T6: otaku wa yoku wakatte masu nante kyuukyuusya no [hito yuu mono.
H6: [un, [un,
K6: [an an,

T7: dakara uti wa moo sugu mon akete,
H7: he,

T8: anoo, husu-[husuma made zenbu hazusite ne, [$######$,
H8: [a, [un,
K8: aa tanka ga ne.
R8: < h h h >

T9: nee, sosite moo, anoo,
K9: uun hairu yoo ni,

T10: kyuukyuusya ni ireru [to sooyuu,
H10: [sorede kyuukyuusya no kata ga kuru to naoru wake?

T11: iya sore [ni noseru desyo? [son toki wa mada wakaranai no [ne.
H11: [un un un, [un un,
K11: [$IYA SOO ZYA NAI$, [< h h h >
R11: [<H H H H H H H>

Translation

T1: yes.
K1: If you leave him without the treatment, will he go to Heaven?

H2: Well, an ambulance usually doesn't come within three minutes, right?

T3: But $MOST OF THE [TIME$ < h > $IT ARRIVES, THAT'S WHY HE IS STILL ALIVE$.
K3: [< H H H H H H >
R3: < H H H H H H H >

T4: [qui-,
H4: [does it?
R4: < H H H H H H >

T5: Well, <H H H H h h > already, w-
H5: < H H H H H H H H H H>
K5: < H H H H H H >
R5: Oh my < H H H H H HH HH>

T6: we already know well where your house is, the ambulance [crew says.
H6: [hmm [hmm
K6: [uh huh

T7: So, I open the gate right away,
H7: ah,

T8: and including slide-[sliding doors, I take down everything [$######$
H8: [uh [huh,
K8: I see,
so a stretcher,

R8: < h h h>

T9: right, and then, well
K9: ahh, so they can enter

T10: once they have him in the ambulance, [they have those,
H10: [and once the ambulance crew has
arrived he recovers?

T11: No, first [in he goes, right? [At that time we still don't know [yet.
H11: [uh huh [uh huh
K11: [$I DON'T THINK SO$, [< h h h >
R11: [<H H H H H H H>

It is interesting to note that the interaction in a situation of collaborative reframing, such as in the examples above, more closely resembles co-constructed playful talk among women (Coates 2007) than talk about troubles as discussed by Jefferson (1984),[5] even though the topic clearly is a serious one. This is possible, I argue, because the serious and painful event is told by the speaker in a different frame that allows for humor and laughter.

An important aspect of quotidian reframing is that the speakers (and collaborating hearers) can reidentify themselves with their "ordinary" or "quotidian" identities in reframed narratives even though the topic of the narrated past experience is psychologically loaded and out of the ordinary. In the reframing in lines A7 to A16 in Extract (1), for example, Akiko presented her regular and familiar identity through a detailed description of a scene that is similar to her regular life with her husband. By presenting a scene from a quotidian perspective, Akiko was able to regain her "normal" identity even though the situation that she was in and was talking about was something out of the ordinary. In a similar fashion, in Extracts (2) and (3), Tamako and her friends enjoy a verbal exchange, even though the topic is the serious medical condition of Tamako's husband. The identity portrayed in those examples is that of a (supposedly dutiful) wife whose quotidian life revolves around daily chores. Because the conversational partners are aware that Akiko's account of being told by her husband to shush was not meant as a complaint to elicit sympathy, and that Tamako did not confuse the ambulance driver with a delivery service, they can understand that both speakers, by changing to a different narrative key, aim at creating a connection to their "normal" or "quotidian" self and, as they are facing difficult changes in their lives, thus try to regain a sense of stability and security.

Regaining a Sense of a "Normal" Self

The extracts discussed above have shown how speakers can talk about past experiences of psychologically tense events by reframing them in a context of everyday life experiences and do so in a way that is enjoyable both to themselves and their conversation partners. In this quotidian framing, the speakers can focus on their identity in ordinary life situations rather than on how their identity would be defined by the serious events being discussed. Apart from being a widow or a wife at her husband's deathbed, for example, the same person is also a woman who has an ordinary daily life. The differing identities coexist, even in conversations about a single topic. A similar point may be made about people who are cared for by others; that is, their identities as care recipients coexist with other identities that may be highlighted in a reframed situation. Extract (4), which is from a 35-minute conversation recorded in a care facility for old people and discussed in the following, illustrates this well.

The interlocutors of this light-hearted conversation are Miwa-san (M) and Shiga-san (S), two relatively healthy female residents and roommates at a care facility in Saitama Prefecture, who received regular visits from a young male researcher (P). At the time of the recording Shiga-san was 73 years old, Miwa-san only 54. Miwa-san had been admitted to the care facility after a stroke a few years prior to the recording. Her case presents a disjunction between chronological age and "functional age" based on physical abilities. The recorded conversation took place while sitting in the hall after breakfast. Miwa-san was coloring a drawing, one of her favorite morning activities, and she did most of the talking, while Shiga-san mainly commented with laughter.

The extract starts with Miwa-san explaining that her drawing portrays Shiga-san happily drinking beer with her (late) husband, adding that she is drawing many hearts on the picture because Shiga-san was so "deeply in love" (*zokkon*) with her husband who was "kind" (*yasasii*) to her. She also suggests that the picture could be displayed at the front door and that Shiga-san might want to keep playing a specific song, the lyrics of which keep repeating the line "my darling, darling husband," although her (dead) husband might complain one day that "it's too noisy" (line M17: *urusa:i nante yuu ka wakannai*).

(4) Conversation at a care facility: A happy couple

M1: kore mite
S1: <HHHHH>
P1: ii desu nee.

M2: Siga-san no o otoosan, hutari de biiru nonde [#
S2: <h> <HHHHH> <H [HH>
P2: [demo nomanai desyo

S3: ee no [nomenai.
P3: zen [zen zenzen nomenai desu ka.

M4: watasi, zenzen nomemasu
S4: <H [HHH>
P4: < [HHH>

M5: nomisugi [ta kara, koo nattyatta.
S5: < [HHH> <HHH>

M6: haatomaaku [ippaikaku. haatomaaku.
S6: < [HHH> < [HHH> <h>
P6: [yasasii desu ne, Miwa-san

M7: Siga-san no otoosan [yasasii mon ne.
S7: < [h> <HHH>
P7: <h>

M8: Siga-san ga zokkon nandamon [ne
S8: < [HHHHH>

M9: [dakara, haatomaaku ippai kaite oitakara ne run run da ne.
S9: <[HHHHH> <HHHH> <hh> <HHHHH>
P9: <h> <h>

M10: run run
S10: <H> <HH>

M11: kore ga dekkaku nareba ne, kazatte [oke n no yo. genkan kara zuutto ne
S11: < [hhh> <Hhhhh>
P11: <h>

P12: ii desu ne.
S12: <HH>

M13: (*imitating Shiga's voice*) otoo-san aisiteru waa
S13: <Hhh>

M14: sorede, tune ni nan dakke, ano uta o nagasite-okeba uti n naka.

M15: watasi no danna sama [ttsute uta o nagasite okeba
S15: < [Hhhhh>

M16: [daizi na danna sama
S16: watasi no [daizi na daizi na <Hhhhh>

M17: sono uti sa, urusa:i nan [te yuu ka wakannai.
S17: < [Hhhhhhh>

Translation

M1: Look at this
S1: <HHHHH>
P1: That's nice

M2: Mrs. Shiga and her husband. They drink beer together [#
S2: <h> <HHHHH> H[<HH>
P2: [but, you don't drink, do you?

S3: No, [I can't.
P3: Not [at all? You can't drink at all?

M4: I can drink at all.
S4: <HHHH>
P4: <HHH>

M5: Because I drank too much [I became like this.
S5: [<HHH> <HHH>

M6: Hearts. [I draw many hearts.
S6: <[HHH> <[HHH> <h>
P6: [You're so kind, Mrs. Miwa.

M7: Mrs. Shiga's husband [is kind, isn't he?
S7: <[h> <HHH>
P7: <h>

M8: Mrs. Shiga is deeply in love with him, [right?
S8: <[HHHHH>

M9: [So, I've drawn lots of heart marks It's happy happy.
S9: <[HHHHH> <HHHH> <hh> <HHHHH>
P9: <h> <h>

M10: Happy happy
S10: <H> <HH>

M11: If it gets bigger, you could display it. All the way from the front door
S11: <hhh> <Hhhhh>
P11: <h>

P12: That's nice.
S12: <HH>

M13: (*imitating Shiga's voice*) I love you
S13: <Hhh>

M14: and, you can always have that song, what's it called, playing in the house

M15: "my dear husband" [If you have that song playing that says that
S15: <[Hhhhh>

M16: [Darling husband
S16: my [Darling, darling <Hhhhh>

M17: One of these days, [(he) might say "Stop it!"
S17: <[Hhhhhhh>

Although what is being verbally disclosed in this extract is not a past experience, there are interesting similarities to the use of quotidian reframing and the phenomenon of layered identities observed in Extracts (1), (2), and (3). The interlocutors share the understanding that Shiga-san loved her husband very much because she liked talking about the wonderful time they had together. Even though both women know that Shiga-san's husband has been dead for some time, Miwa-san's narrative about the couple is carried out in the present tense (lines M7, M8 and M17), as if Shiga-san's husband was still alive and with her. Another noteworthy point is that, while Miwa's drawing depicts Shiga-san drinking beer with her husband, the conversation makes clear that Shiga-san does not drink any alcohol. Miwa-san on the other hand used to drink a lot and, according to her own account, that is why she ended up "like this" (M5). The drawing blends the two different lives that Miwa-san and Shiga-san had before they became residents of the care facility.

Miwa-san's narrative about the drawing is reminiscent of quotidian reframing in that Shiga-san and Miwa-san, while sitting together at a table in a care facility, imagine their former regular life as if it were still present. The description is detailed and contains vivid constructed dialogue as well as laughter, as in the examples of quotidian framing discussed earlier in this chapter. In this example, however, the reframing merges the lives of the two people and thus is more an act of imagination than a presentation of a "real" experience in a different light. Nevertheless, the effect is similar in that the narrator and the participants strategically invoke an identity other than the one that the conversational situation and topic might suggest, thus revealing a complex self-image. It has to be noted here that there was no sign, either in the 35-minute conversation or in the patient records, that Miwa-san was cognitively impaired and therefore might have been confusing past and present. In other parts of the conversation, her comments about real events at the facility and memories of her life in the past gave sufficient proof of this. Further, nobody challenges her description, and in fact the participants join in the story construction.

The conversational narrative in Extract (4) thus could be interpreted as showing that Miwa-san, and possibly also Shiga-san, are attempting to escape from their current reality, or refusing to accept reality, by adhering to the past. Another possible interpretation is that, in the process of accepting the new situation, they are continuing identities from the recent past while making a gradual transition to a not-yet-familiar and externally imposed identity. This may be plausible because, in other parts of the recorded conversation, Miwa-san expressed her resignation to the current situation, admitting that it was her own fault for not taking care of herself. By reframing the current situation to a more familiar one, both participants seem to feel more comfortable; and talking about funny and even silly things could in turn provide a respite and a positive perspective on life. In this sense, the narrative can be interpreted as a way to deal with an additional layer in life without erasing the past, a step toward a new understanding of self, and experiencing transition with a measure of continuity. The reference to their ordinary selves is not a sign of straightforward refusal or unwillingness to change; instead, it provides a secure ground for them to deal with the new situation.

This interpretation is reminiscent of a report (Norrick 2006) on some American women living in a retirement home. These women wanted to show a visitor photographs of their younger selves, as they did not want the visitor to think that they had always been the way they were now. This desire could be interpreted as a negative attitude toward their own old age. However, it can also be understood as a challenge toward the stereotyped characterization of old age and thus a reminder that residents in retirement homes are not just old people with no active role in society but complex individuals, each with a long personal history.

Conclusion

The casual conversations with friends and peers among older Japanese women living independently or in a care facility reveal humor and laughter when the conversation is in a quotidian frame, a frame in which events are depicted from the perspective of an ordinary and familiar situation, regardless of the extraordinariness of the topic or situation. In that way, the moment of the death of one's spouse can be presented from the perspective of a complaint about one's everyday life, just like the recurrent dispatch of an ambulance comes to be described as a delivery service. Likewise, life in a care facility can be reframed to remind the interlocutors of their familiar past lives. In such framing, the speakers and the participants of the conversations can regain their quotidian identities and their understanding of who they are, and they can enjoy laughter in the conversations. Reference to (past) ordinary life and identity can provide familiar ground for people, especially those who are constantly facing the challenges of old age.

These findings carry several implications for communication in elderly care. One is that—as the narratives reframed as quotidian illustrate—there may be several aspects and identities that one person can present. Being a care recipient does not account for the entire person, nor does it erase the identity (or identities) of that person. Another implication is the importance to old people of interacting with friends and peers, verbally or otherwise. The humor and laughter observed in the extracts in this chapter were supported by the sentiment and knowledge shared by the interlocutors and the fostered trust among them. Having opportunities for cultivating friendship appears to be another important ingredient in successful communication among and with older people. While this sounds obvious when considering communication among other age groups, it merits emphasis in the context of eldercare, where many of the interpersonal relationships are defined institutionally on the basis of caregiver and care recipient roles.

The findings further suggest that having relatively lengthy conversations provides a chance for the participants to develop a topic in different aspects, including the quotidian and humorous, even when the topic is as grave and serious as death and illness. Indeed, it could be argued that the humorous sequences presented in this chapter would not have occurred in the first place if the conversations had been shorter.

Talking about painful or psychologically tense topics does not necessarily have only negative effects but can have a positive, almost cathartic function, especially when such topics are developed with humor. Interestingly, this point contrasts with beliefs held by residents and staff members in a U.S. caring facility. Bower (forthcoming), who bases her findings on previous studies (including Bennett 1963; Kaakinen 1992; Hubbard et al. 2003), mentions that topics such as dying, illness, and residents' life before entering a nursing home are considered to be inappropriate. The extracts analyzed in this chapter challenge these findings; they have shown that older adults intentionally and explicitly take up these topics to display multilayered identities in interaction.

Practical Implications

This study advocates the fluidity of roles played by the caregivers (as well as the care recipients). Rather than keeping the rigid division of caregiver and care recipient—or, person in full health vs. person in declining health—adopting various roles suitable for different situations can encourage more satisfying communication. This suggestion is based on the fact that the older adults in my study interact in different frames and present different identities, often choosing to reground themselves in a prior familiar identity. For the purposes of encouraging conversation, caregivers could look for ways to play roles other than those institutionally defined, such as a daughter (see Backhaus, this volume), a friend, or someone who shares the same hobby or interests.

A related point is the importance of remaining aware that each older person has a continuous personal history, which will not be superseded or forgotten in the current situation. Reference to this history may be appreciated by the care recipients, as that would help them to realign themselves with their familiar identity.

Tapping into these various aspects of the care recipients' identity may be facilitated by organizing group gatherings at a facility for both residents and day visitors, which may be used as a resource for new connections (friendships) among the residents. Such friendships are likely to be appreciated by older care recipients at various stages of life-changes and would lead to a more satisfying experience under care.

Notes

[1] A recording of a 35-minute conversation was kindly made available to me by Peter Backhaus. My thanks are also due for the stimulating discussions of the participants of the conference "Communication in Institutional Elderly Care: Cross-Cultural Perspectives," where part of the original version of this chapter was presented. I am grateful to Peter Backhaus and Florian Coulmas for organizing the conference.

[2] On distinctions for different types of discourse, see Chafe (1994).

[3] All speakers' names appearing in this chapter are pseudonyms, except for (Y), which stands for the author's own name.

[4] The "incongruity theory" of humor has been developed and expanded by many scholars, including Bergson (1911 [1899]), Bateson (1953, 2000 [1972]), Giora (1991), Koestler (1964), Norrick (1993, 2003) and Raskin and Attardo (1994).

Although most of these analyses were proposed at a more abstract level or for non-spontaneous humor, such as retold jokes (or "canned jokes"), the basic concept is also manifest and exploited in the conversational narratives in this study. From a related but different point of view, Chafe (2007) proposed "non-seriousness" to be the determining factor behind laughter and humor.

[5] This contrasts with previous findings (Jefferson 1984) that showed that normally only the speaker and not the listeners laughed during talk about troubles, unless there was a buffer topic or a pleasantry involved. The teller and the hearers in the examples quoted in this chapter laugh despite the fact that the related events are not "time-outs" for pleasantries, or "buffer topics" in Jefferson's sense (1984: 351–2). Buffer topics, according to Jefferson, "can consist of jokes and anecdotes associated with the trouble, or quite unrelated matters."

References

Bateson, G. (1953). The position of humor in human communication. In H. von Foerster, (ed.), *Cybernetics, Ninth Conference*, 1–47. New York: Josiah Macy, Jr. Foundation.

—(2000) [1972]. *Steps to An Ecology of Mind.* Chicago, IL: The University of Chicago Press.

Bennett, R. (1963). The meaning of institutional life. *The Gerontologist* 3. 117–25.

Bergson, H. (1911) [1899]. *Laughter: An Essay on the Meaning of the comic.* New York: Macmillan.

Bower, A. R. (Forthcoming). The value of talk: Critical perspectives on studying the speech practices of elderly people in the United States with implications for Japan. In Yoshiko Matsumoto (ed.), *Faces of Aging: The Lived Experiences of the Elderly in Japan.* Stanford, CA: Stanford University Press.

Chafe, W. (1994). *Discourse, Consciousness, and Time: The Flow and Displacement of Conscious Experience in Speaking and Writing.* Chicago, IL: The University of Chicago Press.

—(2007). *The Importance of Not Being Earnest: The Feeling Behind Laughter and Humor.* Amsterdam/Philadelphia, PA: John Benjamins.

Coates, J. (2007). Talk in a play frame: More on laughter and intimacy. *Journal of Pragmatics* 39. 29–49.

Coupland, N., J. Coupland & H. Giles. (1991). *Language, Society and the Elderly: Discourse, Identity and Aging.* Oxford: Basil Blackwell, Inc.

Davis, B. H. (ed.) (2005). *Alzheimer Talk, Text and Context.* New York: Palgrave.

Giora, R. (1991). On the cognitive aspects of the joke. *Journal of Pragmatics* 16. 465–86.

Goffman, E. (1974). *Frame Analysis.* Cambridge, MA: Harvard University Press.

Hamilton, H. E. (1994). *Conversations with an Alzheimer's Patient: An Interactional Sociolinguistics Study.* Cambridge: Cambridge University Press.

Hubbard, G., S. Tester & M. Downs. (2003). Meaningful social interactions between older people in institutional care settings. *Ageing and Society* 23. 99–114.

Jefferson, G. (1984). On the organization of laughter in talk about troubles. In J. M. Atkinson & J. Heritage (eds), *Structures of Social Action*, 346–69. Cambridge; Cambridge University Press.

Kaakinen, J. (1992). Living with silence. *The Gerontologist* 32(2). 258–64.

Koestler, A. 1964. *The Act of Creation.* New York: Macmillan.

Matsumoto, Y. (2005). 'We'll be dead by then!'—Comical self-disclosure by elderly Japanese women. In M. Ettlinger, N. Fleischer & M. Park-Doob (eds.), *Proceedings of the 30th Annual Meeting of the Berkeley Linguistics Society*, 268–79. Berkeley, CA: Berkeley Linguistics Society.

—(2008). Discourse of the elderly from the speaker's point of view. In Junko Mori and Amy S. Ohta (eds), *Japanese Applied Linguistics: Discourse and Social Perspectives*, 188–210. Continuum International Publishing Group: New York.

—(2009). Dealing with changes—Humorous self-disclosure by elderly Japanese women. *Ageing and Society* 29 (Issue 6: Discourse, identity and change in mid-to-late life: Interdisciplinary perspectives on language and ageing), 929–52.

—(forthcoming). Painful to playful: Quotidian frames in the conversational discourse of older Japanese women. *Language in Society* 40(5).

Norrick, N. R. (1993). *Conversational Joking.* Bloomington, IN: Indiana University Press.

—(2003). Issues in conversational joking. *Journal of Pragmatics* 35. 1333–59.

—(2006). *Narrative Construction of Multiple Identities by Older Adults.* Paper presented at the Sociolinguistics Symposium 16, University of Limerick, Ireland, 6–8 July.

Raskin, V. & S. Attardo. (1994). Non-literalness and non-bona-fide in language. *Pragmatics and Cognition* 2. 31–69.

Ryan, E. B., M. L. Hummert & L. Boich. (1995). Communication predicaments of aging: Patronizing behavior toward older adults. *Journal of Language and Social Psychology* 14(1–2). 144–66.

Tannen, D. (1979). What's in a frame?—Surface evidence for underlying expectations. In Roy Freedle (ed.), *New Directions in Discourse Processing*, 137–81. Norwood, NJ: Ablex.

—(1989). *Talking Voices: Repetition, Dialogue, and Imagery in Conversational Discourse.* New York: Cambridge University Press.

Chapter 9

At the Intersection of Art, Alzheimer's Disease, and Discourse: Talk in the Surround of Paintings

Heidi E. Hamilton

Guide: *It's interesting these- these lovely lovely movements in the- in this image. With the- the joining of- of arms. Wonder when this is meant to be. These hairstyles and tiny little eyebrows- pointy shoes.*

Katherine: *Well when I was a teenager we bought- we called them ballerina skirts. They were very popular.*

Guide: *Ah.*

Katherine: *We wore several petticoats underneath.*

—Excerpt from museum tour viewing
Latin American Grand Final by John Brack (1969)

Introduction

Imagine yourself standing in front of a large oil painting, staring up at two dancing couples in a "blaze of neon pinks, stinging reds and sharp thrusts of black" (Grishin 2002). The numbers 33 and 5 tacked to the back of the men's black suits, coupled with the judge standing off to the side, suggest a dance competition. A glance at the oil painting's title, *Latin American Grand Final*, confirms your guess. You turn again toward the painting. What captures your attention? The jolting colors? The full skirts? The angular turn of the head? Do memories of high school dances pop into your mind? Do you find yourself imagining what it would be like to be an elegant dancer? Do you wonder about the relationship between the dance partners? It is this interrelationship between thoughts translated into talk and works of art that occupies us in this chapter, but within a specific context: that of specially designed art museum tours for individuals with Alzheimer's disease. Before we proceed in our exploration of these connections, we need first to provide some background information regarding how language is affected by Alzheimer's disease, and why one might be interested in pursuing a study of this connection within the environment of an art museum.

All individuals with Alzheimer's disease gradually lose their ability to communicate as the disease progresses. Early investigations identified that problems in these areas were due less to disorders on the phonological level (sound system) and the morphosyntactic level (ways in which words and sentences are constructed) than to difficulties on the semantic and pragmatic levels (Bayles and Kaszniak 1987; Kempler 1984). Because of their basically well-formed sentence structure, many of the inappropriate or irrelevant utterances that are characteristic of the language used by early to moderate-stage Alzheimer's patients do not appear out of the ordinary in isolation, but only when heard within their larger discourse context in pursuit of some interactional goal (for more details, see Hamilton 1994a, 1994b).

Building on foundational work that characterizes these linguistic problems as they relate to the production and comprehension of discourse, scholars have begun to understand how these linguistic difficulties relate to issues of self-identity in everyday life (Davis 2005; Hamilton 1996, 2000; Sabat 2001). These interests link up with discussions in the literature outside of linguistics that speak of the identity crises, loss of self, and profound changes in personality (see Cohen and Eisdorfer 1986; Kitwood 1988; Sabat and Harré 1992; Shenk 2005) that accompany the disease.

The vast majority of sociolinguistic work on discursive identity construction has focused on the ways in which people tell narratives of personal experience, arguing that narrative choices can reveal much about how narrators see themselves and how they wish to be seen by those listening to them (see especially De Fina et al. 2006). To illuminate the relationship between narrative production and identity, Schiffrin (1996: 199) uses a powerful visual image, that of a "self-portrait."

> Telling a story provides a self-portrait: a linguistic lens through which to discover peoples' own (somewhat idealized) views of themselves as situated in a social structure. The verbalization and textual structure of a story [. . .] combines with its content, and with its local and global contexts of production, to provide a view of self that can be either challenged or validated by an audience.

However, given the increasingly severe memory problems that accompany linguistic decline as the disease progresses, one wonders whether individuals with Alzheimer's disease can recount personal experiences in the form of narratives at all; and, if they can, whether these narratives comprise enough linguistic detail to do meaningful identity work (i.e, whether the narrator is seen as self-confident, caring, deferential, etc.). In an effort to explore these issues within everyday conversations involving an individual with Alzheimer's disease (Hamilton 2008) I found, first, that the vast majority (85%) of the communication referred not to memories or abstract thoughts, but to people, objects, and actions within the immediate physical environment—a finding that provides additional empirical evidence for the "context-boundedness" identified in early examinations of Alzheimer's patients (Appell, Kertesz and Fisman 1982; Obler 1981). Second, the few narratives that *were* told were invariably triggered by an object in the here and now. And, third, the linguistically constructed storyworlds lacked vividness due to a high use of pronouns and semantically "empty" words, such as "place," "thing" "make" and "do."

Running parallel to this line of scholarship on Alzheimer's disease, discourse, and identity is a robust movement in innovative programming at the intersection of arts and Alzheimer's disease. Recently created scholarly societies, journals, and conferences facilitate investigations regarding the effectiveness of creative expression therapy in a variety of artistic domains, including music, visual arts, and the writing of poetry and short stories (for an overview, see Zeisel 2009; also Ryan and Schindel Martin, this volume). Proponents claim that these multisensory experiences that focus on personhood are especially good at promoting the social and creative well-being of Alzheimer's patients. Because language is an observable representation of individuals' mental activities, rigorous linguistic analyses would arguably provide powerful evidence of the cognitive and social effects of such programs on participants. To my knowledge, however, no linguist has studied the discourse produced by participants in such artistic endeavors.[1] My long-standing interest in the relationship of language to Alzheimer's disease, coupled with a personal interest in and awareness of the critical importance of art in social life, energized me to address this gap.

Based on my earlier findings regarding the close connection between objects in the physical environment and narratives told in Alzheimer discourse (i.e., that physical objects in the immediate environment seem to trigger memories that are then displayed in personal experience narratives), I decided to begin my exploration of Alzheimer's disease and the arts within a *visual* arts program rather than a music or writing program that would involve no such physical triggers. I sought a meeting with John Zeisel, President of Hearthstone Alzheimer Care in Massachusetts, who has designed and carried out special tours for individuals with Alzheimer's disease at the Museum of Modern Art (MOMA) in New York City and the Louvre in Paris (see Zeisel 2009: 87–103). Zeisel approaches these tours with a missionary's zeal. He describes his motivation as follows:

> When art is a profound part of the everyday flow of life for people living with Alzheimer's, it offers a vibrant and extraordinary dimension [. . .] Because people living with Alzheimer's tend to express what they think and feel at the moment, they are natural artists and natural audiences for artistic expression. (Zeisel 2009: 81)

Zeisel's tours have met with great success (see Blakemore 2006; Kennedy 2005), with proponents claiming that the language and affect of individuals with Alzheimer's disease improved during and after the tours where the individuals could interact with paintings in a low-stress, unhurried environment. This evidence is compelling, but so far anecdotal (Kennedy 2005):

> It [the art therapy] seems to be working, though no one knows exactly how. While extensive research has been conducted on the effects of music and performing arts on brain function [. . .] there has been comparatively little work done in the visual arts. What

exists mostly is a stockpile of anecdotal evidence, encouraging but murky.

As a result of our discussions, Zeisel invited me to become involved as the only linguist in a pilot interdisciplinary study entitled "A pilot evaluation of access to art gallery tours for people with dementia" at the National Gallery of Australia in New South Wales (see McPherson et al. 2009). I was asked to design a linguistic methodology that would be able to evaluate effects of the museum project on participants as evidenced in the discourse produced within these interactions. Findings based on this methodology would then complement findings based on other instruments, including assessments of memory and affect, pre- and post-intervention questionnaires, and focus group interviews involving the individuals with Alzheimer's disease, their caregivers, and gallery guides. The first phase of that effort is reported here. It is my hope that this methodology may be utilized not only to evaluate these museum-based activities, but to assist in both the design and the execution of new ones. These insights may even extend beyond the walls of the museum to relate to any activity whose success may be measured by the quantity and quality of the conversational interaction it engenders.

In what follows, I first characterize the participants and interactions involved in the pilot study and outline the assumptions that guided my analytical decisions. Next, I identify and illustrate coding decisions as related to the discourse produced by the visitors with Alzheimer's disease (both quantitative and qualitative analyses) as well as to the discourse environment within which this discourse emerged. I then apply the coding system to the museum tour interactions, highlighting important findings of this application. In closing, I discuss these findings, propose next steps in the analysis, and outline various implications of this project for practice.

Characterization of Participants and Recorded Museum Tour Interactions

The study reported in this chapter is based on transcriptions of video recordings of twelve small-group art gallery tours designed for sixteen individuals with Alzheimer's disease (eight individuals at an early stage and another eight at a more advanced stage of the disease) who were led by specially trained guides at the National Gallery of Australia in New South Wales, Australia. This special design included deliberations regarding the purpose of the tours and the way in which related activities would support that purpose. Guides were asked to consider a shift in focus from teaching about the paintings to "encourag[ing] the participants to express what they see and feel about the art" (Zeisel 2009: 98). Each group of eight was divided into smaller groups that took part in six weekly one-hour tours, each time viewing and discussing on average four works of art. Twelve of

Table 9.1. Works of art viewed during museum tours 1, 3, and 6

Tour number	Works of art viewed and discussed (in order of viewing)
1	*The Flapper* by Margaret Preston (1925) http://artsearch.nga.gov.au/Detail.cfm?IRN=74868 *The Sunday Stroll* by Robert Dickerson (1960) http://artsearch.nga.gov.au/Detail.cfm?IRN=141620 *Interior in Yellow* by Grace Cossington Smith (1962/1964) http://artsearch.nga.gov.au/Detail.cfm?IRN=45746 *Her Father's Servant* by Julie Dowling (1999) http://artsearch.nga.gov.au/Detail.cfm?IRN=12869
3	*Four Panels for a Screen* by Grace Cossington Smith 1928 http://www.nga.gov.au/exhibition/cossingtonsmith/Detail.cfm?IRN=115741 *Reflected Bride*: Arthur Boyd 1958 http://artsearch.nga.gov.au/Detail.cfm?IRN=12774 *Feathered Fence* by Rosalie Gascoigne (1979) http://artsearch.nga.gov.au/Detail.cfm?IRN=177908 *Suddenly the Lake* by Rosalie Gascoigne, 1995 http://www.roslynoxley9.com.au/artists/15/Rosalie_Gascoigne/547/40063/
6	*Spirit of the Plains* by Sydney Long, 1914 http://cs.nga.gov.au/Detail.cfm?IRN=82425 *Fireplace Surround and Mantel* by Robert Prenzel (1910) http://artsearch.nga.gov.au/Detail.cfm?IRN=30130&PICTAUS=TRUE *The Flapper* by Margaret Preston (1925) http://artsearch.nga.gov.au/Detail.cfm?IRN=74868 *Christian Waller with Baldur, Undine and Siren at Fairy Hills*: Napier Waller 1932 http://cs.nga.gov.au/Detail.cfm?IRN=49895 *Latin American Grand Final* by John Brack (1969) http://cs.nga.gov.au/Detail.cfm?IRN=109694

these twenty-four tours (weeks 1, 3, and 6 for each tour group) were recorded on video and audio.

The first phase of the coding process centered on three of these twelve tours that included three visitors with early-stage Alzheimer's disease, Esther, Emma, and Katherine (all pseudonyms) with two museum guides. Works of art that served as a springboard for verbal interaction within each tour are listed in Table 9.1, along with the associated URL to allow interested readers to view them.

Each museum tour was transcribed[2] in its entirety and divided into tour segments I call "stops" that corresponded to the physical movement and content discussions of the individuals as they paused on the tour to view and discuss individual works of art. The three tours contained eleven stops that focused on thirteen works of art because, in two instances, the tour group discussed two works of art from the same location in the museum.

Guiding Assumptions

Before proceeding to the specifics of the linguistic methodology, it is important to take a moment to outline the assumptions that guided my decisions regarding where and how to begin to code the language used within the turns produced at the stops within the museum.

First, I assume that the discourse produced by individual museum visitors will vary quantitatively and qualitatively (see, for example, studies in Davis 2005), both within single tours and across the tours. Further, since these are all multi-party interactions, variation can be expected in the ways in which turns-at-talk are distributed (see Heritage 1997; Sacks et al. 1974). Sociolinguistic studies of discourse and Alzheimer's disease have shown variability in discourse production to be related (at least in part) to aspects of the discourse context (see, e.g., Ramanathan 1997), just as is the case for healthy interlocutors. The contexts within which the museum tour discourse is produced need, therefore, to be carefully examined for evidence of possible influence of interlocutors (e.g., guides or other visitors), physical surroundings (including here the artwork being discussed), type of speech event (e.g., lecture, discussion, small talk, etc.), and the framing (Goffman 1974) of the event, as well as the degree to which the interaction is constructed as institutional vs. everyday discourse (Heritage 1997).

Second, in terms of *quantitative* variation, I assume that relatively extensive discourse production by museum visitors can serve as evidence of successful programming. Ritchhart's thoughts on the cultivation of a culture of thinking in museums, although meant to guide school groups, highlight the importance of creating an environment in which "cognition, affect, social context, and the environment are fully integrated [. . . and] the group's collective as well as individual thinking is *valued, visible,* and *actively promoted* as part of the ongoing experience of all group members" (Ritchhart 2007: 139, emphasis original). Inherent in all these considerations is the important role that speaking plays. Social activities, such as the museum tours that are at the center of this study, provide important opportunities for individuals to move from the thought processes of the single mind to "making thinking visible" (Perkins 2003) through extended discussion and sharing of ideas and opinions. From a linguistic point of view, this move from thought to speech within a group is methodologically useful in that extensive turns-at-talk—in contrast to minimal responses, such as "yes" or "I agree"—provide language clues regarding possible effects of the art program on their speakers.

Third, in terms of *qualitative* variation, I assume that museum visitors of any kind (not just those with Alzheimer's disease) can select from among a large repertoire of appropriate responses when engaging with art, including at least the following: describing aspects of the work of art, evaluating it, interpreting it, reacting viscerally to it, judging it, connecting it to other works of art (visual or otherwise), telling a story or going off on a flight of fancy based on the world suggested by it, and recounting personal or general memories sparked by it (see Housen 2001; Tishman and Palmer 2006; Zeisel 2009). Happily, this range of appropriate responses allows for individuals with different levels of severity of Alzheimer's disease to participate actively in museum tours. For example, individuals who have more extensive memory loss and are perhaps more bound to the context of the "here and now" can participate by describing what they see in the work of art or commenting on how it makes them feel. Others at an earlier stage of the disease whose memories are relatively more intact may be able to connect personal and/or general memories to aspects of the works of art, allowing for the kind of identity construction discussed by Schiffrin (1996) and others.

Finally, I assume that a lively turn-exchange among museum visitors can be understood as an indicator of successful arts programming. In addition to the importance placed on what Leinhart and Crowley (2002) call "conversational elaboration" (as cited in Ritchhart 2007: 148) in which "greater detail, connections and explanations emerge in the group talk of visitors as a result of their experience in the museum," other educational researchers (Erickson n.d.; Lazarus and Smith 1988) have used the term "hot cognition" (Abelson 1963) to characterize the lively discursive exchange of ideas that combines emotion with cognition and contrasts markedly with more subdued passive "reception" of knowledge. Devising a way to characterize the turn exchange during these tours is critical to the assessment of the degree of institutional quality of the discourse in general. For example, characterizations of institutional discourse by Heritage (1997) clearly indicate that interactions comprising questions asked by tour guides followed immediately by visitors' responses are more representative of institutional discourse than, for example, museum visitors' initiation of engagement with each other, as more control over the interaction is being exerted by the institutional representative in the first instance (regarding questions and control, see Ainsworth-Vaughn 1998).

Discourse Coding Decisions

Guided by the assumptions outlined above, I turned my attention first to the discourse produced by the visitors—both quantitatively and qualitatively—within the museum tours. In order to provide evidence as to the sheer amount of talk produced by the visitors within this set of transcribed interactions, I first examined the visitors' discourse in terms of the length of each turn-at-talk. To this end, I identified each turn as: (1) a minimal response, (2) a single grammatical clause, or (3) more than one grammatical clause. Illustrations of these categories can be found in Table 9.2.

Table 9.2. Quantitative coding of visitor turns-at-talk

Length of visitor turn-at-talk	**Illustration from the museum tours**
(1) minimal response	*Oh my!*
(2) single clause	*It's quite lovely.*
(3) more than one clause	*Well when I was a teenager we bought . . . we called them ballerina skirts. They were very popular.*

Next, I examined visitors' turns-at-talk from categories (2) and (3) of the quantitative analysis (turns-at-talk comprising single clauses and more than one clause) and determined the qualitative type of visitor turn. Because of the project's focus on the connection between speakers' identity and the narratives they produce (and the identified challenge in locating sufficient narrative utterances produced by individuals with Alzheimer's disease due to memory problems), I decided it would be important to distinguish turns-at-talk that recounted a memory (whether personal or general) from turns-at-talk that did not. I based my coding decisions on Chafe (1994: 210–211) who understands talk as an outward linguistic display of the human consciousness and its "ability to focus, not just on the immediate environment, but also on remembered and imagined experience." That is, a speaker's consciousness can remain in what Chafe terms the "immediate mode" and *perceive, act,* and *evaluate* people, objects, and actions in their immediate surroundings or it can move to a "displaced mode" and *remember* or *imagine* people, objects, and actions in times and/or places not in the here and now. Table 9.3 provides illustrations of each type of qualitative coding determination made.

Turning from an exclusive focus on the discourse produced by the museum visitors to the discourse environment within which the visitors' discourse emerged, I focused on the turn exchange system. Recall from the discussion of assumptions above that a lively exchange of turns involving visitors (in contrast with guide questions followed by visitor responses) can serve as a barometer both of visitor interest and engagement and of the level of institutional quality of the discourse produced as part of these museum tours. To this end, each visitor turn-at-talk identified in the transcribed tour interactions was given the designation of turn 0 (zero). For each such instance, I

Table 9.3. Qualitative coding of visitor turns-at-talk (based on Chafe 1994)

Qualitative category	Associated actions	Transcript illustrations
1. Immediate mode	Perceive	*There's quite a lot of candles on that cake.*
	Act	*I agree with you.*
	Evaluate	*It looks warm and comfortable.*
2. Displaced mode	Remember: general	*They didn't wear mini-dresses in those days.*
	Remember: personal	*We lived in a big old house.*
	Imagine	*There might have been bad news in the letter.*

Table 9.4. Coding of "turn −1" as part of turn exchange system analysis

Type of participant producing a −1 utterance	Discourse illustrations from tours ('turn −1' is indicated by an → on the left)	
(1) Another visitor	Assertion	
	→ −1. Esther:	I don't know that's a chair.
	0. Emma:	It IS a chair.
	Question	
	→ −1. Katherine:	Do you remember the sack dress came into fashion—that was in the- the- in the early forties?
	0. Esther:	I had one. I had to get one.
(2) A guide	Assertion	
	→ −1. Guide:	I agree with you, Esther.
	0. Esther:	Yes, they grow up very quickly.
	Question	
	→ −1. Guide:	Is this a room where she spent a lot of time?
	0. Esther:	Yes, I think so.

identified the utterance that immediately preceded it in the transcript and termed it "turn −1." I then determined what type of participant (guide or visitor) produced the turn −1 and whether it was a question or an assertion. Table 9.4 provides illustrations of the turn −1 coding according to speaker.

With these coding decisions illustrated, I turn now to the application of the methodology to the discourse that unfolded within the 11 stops on the three museum tours.

Application of the Coding System to the Museum Tours

Over the course of all three recorded museum tours, the visitors took 661 turns-at-talk: 248 during the first tour, 201 during the third tour, and 212 during the sixth tour. As shown in Table 9.5, quantitative analyses revealed that the largest proportion of turns-at-talk comprised a single clause (41%) followed next by minimal responses (34%) and more than one clause (25%). In other words, when visitors took the initiative to talk, two-thirds of the time their turns contributed to propositions being discussed; one-third of the time, their turns did little more than display simple (dis)agreement or provide other very minimal evaluation.

Of the 435 (66%) turns-at-talk that were at least one clause long, in 94 (22%) instances the visitor recounted a memory. Of these 94 utterances, 48 were general memories; 46 were personal ones. When these findings are considered within the full interactional context of the museum tour (i.e., including the many visitor turns that comprised only minimal responses), they show that 14% of visitor turns-at-talk on average recounted a memory of some kind; 7% recounted a personal experience memory. In this category, individual stops within the museum varied widely, ranging from the discussion of *Sunday Stroll,* in which not a single visitor recounted a memory, to the discussion of *Latin American Grand Final,* in which a remarkable 74% of visitor turns referenced a memory. If it is indeed one goal of these museum programs to spark visitors' memories and to encourage group discussion of past cultural products and practices, it is necessary to focus on the relative importance of the images themselves as well as on the guides' use of language to facilitate or hinder such communicative time travel.

Turning to the discourse context of the visitors' turns-at-talk (see Table 9.6), 90% (or 595) of utterances leading to visitors' turns were produced by the guides as contrasted with only 10% (or 66) being produced by the other visitors. This finding highlights the highly institutional nature of the museum tours (see Heritage 1997) as contrasted with a more fluid conversational interaction that would involve

Table 9.5. Length of visitors' turns-at-talk during three museum tours

Minimal responses	***n* = 226 (34%)**
Single clause	*n* = 270 (41%)
More than one clause	*n* = 165 (25%)
Total:	*n = 661 (100%)*

Table 9.6. Analysis of the turn exchange system in three museum tours

Guide as speaker	**595 utterances (90%)** 454 (76%) were assertions 141 (24%) were questions
Another visitor as speaker	**66 utterances (10%)** 56 (85%) were assertions 10 (15%) were questions

relatively equal contributions by all participants. Interestingly, in both cases, the institutional nature of the interaction appears at first blush to be blunted somewhat by the fact that the visitors' turns-at-talk were significantly more likely to be preceded by assertions than questions; a turn exchange system made up of assertions followed by other assertions is characteristic of a sharing of ideas and opinions in contrast with the more traditional educational discourse frame of questions followed by responses. Upon closer examination, many of the assertions made by the guides turned out to be in the form of "I wonder X" that carried interrogative force even though they arguably did not "require" responses (Schegloff and Sacks 1973) in the same way that questions would have. Such findings point to the challenges faced by guides who downplay their expert status in attempts to nurture visitor contributions.

This coding system can offer guidance in the evaluation of existing art access programs as well as in the construction of new activities that involve a discourse environment that encourages (i) more extensive (and fewer minimal) responses by visitors, (ii) more responses that contain memories by visitors, and (iii) more back-and-forth talk among visitors (not just responses to guides). To this end, information on *average* communicative behavior can be used to identify interactions related to specific works of art that either "overperform" or "underperform" vis-à-vis these averages (see Table 9.7).

Information in Table 9.7 indicates that the following three stops of eleven were most successful: *Flapper* in terms of the amount of talk that the visitors produced, *Latin American Grand Final* in terms of the amount of reminiscing that the visitors did, and *Interior in Yellow* in

Table 9.7. Average communicative behavior by visitors during eleven stops

Behavior	Percentage and range (of turns)	Two 'overperforming' stops	Two 'underperforming' stops
Average percentage of visitor turns longer than one clause	25% (165 of 661) Range: 17–51%	*Flapper* (51%) *Latin American Grand Final* (32%)	*Four Panels for a Screen* (17%) *My Father's Servant* (18%)
Average percentage of minimal responses by visitors	34% (266 of 661) Range: 13–48%	*Flapper* (13%) *Reflected Bride* (28%)	*Feathered Fence* (48%) *Four Panels for a Screen* (45%)
Average percentages of visitor turns that recounted memories	22% (94 of 435) Range: 0–74%	*Latin American Grand Final* (74%) *Flapper* (69%)	*Sunday Stroll* (0%) *Reflected Bride* (2%)
Average percentage of visitor responses that immediately followed other visitor responses	10% (66 of 661) Range: 0–22%	*Interior in Yellow* (22%) *Sunday Stroll* (21%)	*Spirit of the Plains* (0%) *Four Panels for a Screen* (2%)

terms of the amount of dialogue produced among the visitors. Details related to each of these paintings follow, along with a brief extract of the discourse at each stop to put these findings into its authentic context.

Most Successful Stop in Terms of Length of Visitors' Turns-At-Talk

During the time spent in front of *Flapper*, visitors took 45 turns-at-talk, 23 (51%) of which were more than a clause in length and only 6 (13%) of which were classified as minimal responses. These percentages contrasted sharply with averages of 25% and 34%, respectively, for a first place ranking out of all eleven stops and indicate a high level of communicative engagement. To accentuate the differences, if the visitors had produced turns at the average rate, only 11 (not 23) of their turns-at-talk would have been longer than a clause in length and 15 (not 6) would have been minimal responses. Extract (1) illustrates the kind of extensive communication produced by the museum visitors at the *Flapper* stop on the tour.

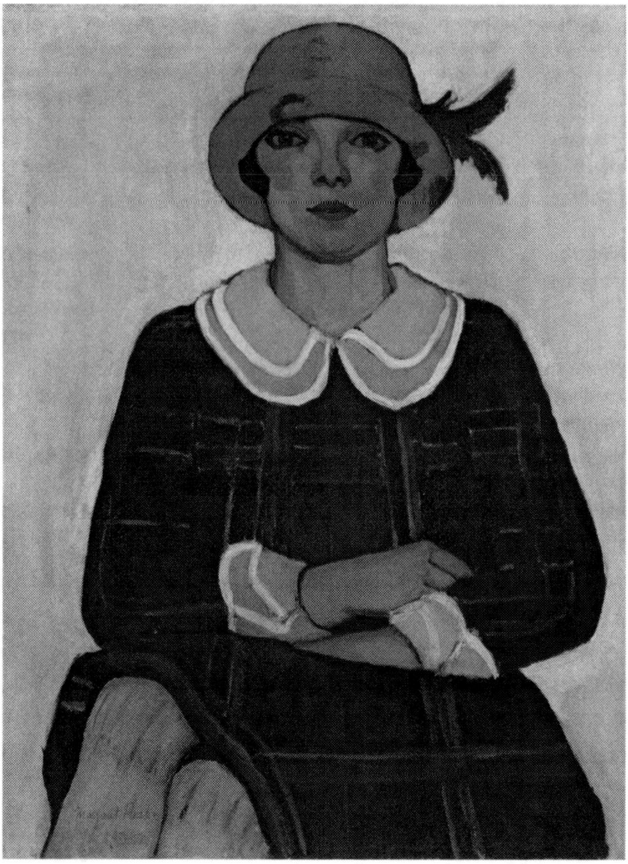

(1) Viewing *Flapper*

1.	Katherine:	They didn't wear mini-dresses in those days.
2.	Guide:	In the 1920s. Yeah. Hmmm.
3.	Esther:	I think they'd like to but they weren't allowed to.
		[*laughter*]
4.	Esther:	Correct?
5.	Katherine:	An- and the clothes were rather shapeless.
6.	Guide:	Yeah. Yeah.
7.	Katherine:	Do you mean this- do you remember the sack dress came into
8.		fashion? That was in the- in the early forties?
9.	Esther:	I had one. I had to get one. The sack was like a sack, no shape to
10.		it at all. Just hung. Called the sack look.
11.	Guide:	Doesn't sound all that fun. I think we all need a bit more contours.

12. Katherine: We went through a depression, and a war, and everything
13. was austere.
14. Guide: Yeah. Yeah, exactly, Katherine. What about this lady here?
15. What do you think she- Is she austere in her dress or=
16. Katherine: =Well, she'd be, to
17. look at her, quite dressy.

Besides the discussion at this stop of the sack dress and the *zeitgeist* that surrounded it, the visitors' extended turns-at-talk had to do with a visitor's mother (visitor-initiated), the feather on the hat (guide-initiated), detachable collar and cuffs (visitor-initiated), colored stockings in the 1960s and 1970s (visitor-initiated), World War II (visitor-initiated), and a comparison of the treatment of children then and now (visitor-initiated).

Most Successful Stop in terms of Visitors' Recounting of Memories

During the time spent in front of *Latin American Grand Final*,[3] visitors took 80 turns-at-talk, 59 (74%) of which recounted a memory, for a first place ranking out of all 11 stops on the 3 tours. This percentage (74%) contrasted sharply with the average of 22% across all 11 stops. To accentuate this distinction, if the visitors had recounted memories at the average rate, only 18 (not 59) of their turns-at-talk would have contained memories. Extract (2) illustrates the talk at this stop.

(2) Viewing *Latin American Grand Final*

1. Guide: Were you- did you- either of you dance in- in this way? Were
2. you=
3. Esther: =Yes. We danced but uh=
4. Katherine: =We used to go dance about three
5. times a week!
6. Guide: I see.
7. Katherine: Doug was out, I think ( ).
8. Guide: And were you the center of attention?
9. Katherine: Mm not really.
10. Esther: I um I did the ballet and tapping. My sister was a very good
11. ballroom dancer. But when you learn ballet and tap you're

12.		never good as a ballroom dancer. The movements are
13.		different. And um, so I was the ballet girl and ( ) did the
14.		ballroom.

Memories recounted by visitors at this stop that extended beyond those related to ballroom and ballet dancing included: fashion as a teenager, personal wedding, husband in the navy, daughter in sports, and hairdos in the past. Of these, a visitor initiated all except for the conversation about hairdos.

Most Successful Stop in terms of Visitor-Visitor Dialogue

During the time spent in front of *Interior in Yellow,* visitors took 73 turns-at-talk, 16 of which (22%) immediately followed another visitor's turn-at-talk, for a first place ranking out of all 11 stops on the three tours. This percentage contrasted with the average of 10% and indicates a relatively high level of engagement among visitors. To accentuate this distinction, if the visitors had interacted at the average rate, only 7 (not 16) of their turns-at-talk would have been in response to another visitor's turn. Extract (3) illustrates the kind of lively back-and-forth among visitors that took place at the *Interior in Yellow* stop on the tour.

Prior to the interaction represented in Extract (3), the guide had introduced the painting and its artist when she asked the visitors, "How does this room make you feel when you look at it?" to which Katherine replied, "It's busy" followed immediately by Emma's agreement "It's very busy!"

(3) Viewing *Interior in Yellow*

1.	Guide:	Yes, Katherine, I agree- that it's very busy=
2.	Emma:	=but it's you know=
3.	Esther:	=I
4.		think it's a very tiny room.
5.	Guide:	Is it?
6.	Esther:	A very tiny room.
7.	Emma:	But it looks warm and comfortable.

8 Guide: It's- it's busy. It IS a tiny room and I like that comment. It is,
9. because as Grace, as her life went on, her world became more into
10. it. And so it IS a tiny room.
11. Visitors: Oh [choral]
12. Guide: And it FEELS like a tiny room=
13. Esther: =yes, yes=
14. Emma: =but it can't be THAT
15. tiny because of the- the little (?). I mean you've only got half of it,
16. you know, so obviously there's more to it than that.
17. Guide: Yes, there's only a section of it.
18. Esther: Yes but I still feel that the room is a tiny room.

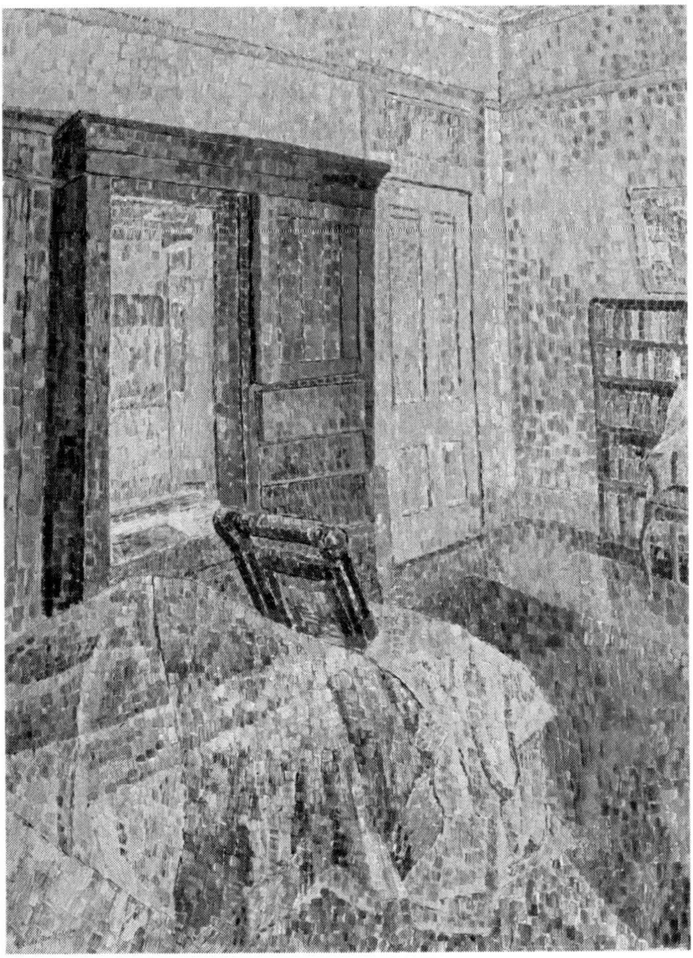

The subsequent interaction at this stop included dialogue regarding visitors' emotional responses to the painting (e.g., intimate, happy, comfortable), identification of details in the painting (e.g., chair, bookshelf), and characterization of the painting's colors (e.g., vibrant, warm). Before moving on to the final painting of the day, the guide asked, "Would you like to live in this room?"—a question that sparked both positive and fervent negative responses ("too messy", "too much", "too colorful") from the visitors.

Discussion

What can we make of the findings above? As had been assumed, significant variation occurred in the language produced by individuals in a small tour group as it made its way through the National Gallery of Australia, stopping to talk at 11 different locations during three weekly one-hour tours. Coding decisions in this first phase of the study focused attention on the length of the visitors' turns-at-talk, whether memories were recounted in these turns, and whether these turns immediately followed turns by other visitors or by the guides. These communicative behaviors were selected for coding based on literature regarding best practices and allowed for an examination of the relative proportions of these communicative behaviors at each stop along the tour.

By comparing individual percentages with average behaviors across all stops, I was able to identify the most successful stop in each category, *Flapper, Latin American Grand Final,* and *Interior in Yellow,* respectively. If the goal of such arts-based programs is to offer individuals with Alzheimer's disease opportunities for engagement, both with a new subject matter (i.e., works of art) and with each other in a social situation, then the contexts related to the three stops mentioned just above can be held up as examples of best practices. Clearly, though, given the complexity of the language used in these tours, the work has just begun. Two key questions arise: What next steps need to be taken as the study moves into its second phase? What recommendations can be derived from these first phase findings for the design, execution, and evaluation of other such arts-based activities?

In response to the first question, phase two will need to move beyond the mere characterization of turns-at-talk and turn exchange to disentangle the relative effects of various aspects of these interactional contexts. Accordingly, phase two will expand on the work reported in this chapter in the following ways:

(1) Since phase one focused on the variation in discourse produced by only one small group of visitors as these visitors viewed different works of art, phase two will hold individual works of art constant and examine variation in discourse about them as produced by different visitors (including individuals living with more advanced stages of Alzheimer's disease).

(2) Additionally, phase two will focus on aspects of the turn exchange system by revisiting the set of turns −1 to determine whether any associations exist between types of turns −1 (assertions, types of questions) and the quantity or quality of subsequent visitor turns (e.g., "Do yes-no questions inhibit responses by visitors in contrast with wh-questions?").

(3) Finally, phase two will include more detailed linguistic analysis of visitor turns—including analysis of affect, and agentive and epistemic stance—in order to study possible shifts over time in visitors' sense of self. These shifts can occur in the here-and-now aspects of the discourse as well as in the representations of self in recounted memories and/or short narratives (e.g., "What emotions are the speakers displaying—now and in the represented past?," "Are they taking control of the situation—now and in the represented past?" and "How certain are they of what they are saying—now and in the represented past?"). Linguistic analyses of the visitor-visitor dialogue will aim to identify ways in which individuals with Alzheimer's disease accomplish joint meaning-making and display affect, as well as agentive and epistemic stance, when expressing opinions and arguing for particular points of view.

Practical Implications

The implications of this study, in combination with findings and discussions regarding educational opportunities in museums by Zeisel (2009), Ritchhart (2007), Leinhardt and Knutson (2004), Housen (2001) and Housen and Yenawine (2001), are many.

The study's emphasis on extended discourse on the part of museum visitors should serve as a guide for new and existing programs within museums. For those with existing programs, "listening in on" communication that takes place in the surround of museum works of art (or even recording, transcribing, and studying it) helps to identify whether the activity is having the kind of communicative effect that was anticipated. Thus works of art may be separated by types of responses that they tend to receive from visitors; guides may be able to reflect on the role their language use is playing in encouraging or discouraging visitor responses; and programs may be able to track changes in visitor behavior over time, as a possible indication of learning, or of becoming more comfortable with the activity. Furthermore, attempts can be made to minimize the percentage of visitors' minimal responses to guides and to other visitors, while encouraging the recounting of memories and the elevation of the peer-peer communication that is indicative of "hot cognition."

Those interested in beginning an arts program for individuals with Alzheimer's disease—whether within a museum or adapted for use in an assisted living center, senior center or for in-home care[4]—will find guidance below regarding both the design and the execution of such activities. Implications include: (i) selection of works of art, (ii) time allocation, (iii) size and constitution of the group, and (iv) discussion routines used by the tour guides.

Selection of Works of Art

Zeisel (2009: 90) emphasizes the importance of choosing works of art that "elicit the cognitive strengths of participants" and recommends a selection process that involves the expected tour participants *before* they arrive in the museum. Individuals can be presented with reproductions (museum store postcards or posters) of possible works of art and, through discussions, end up selecting the art to be included in specific tours. Findings by Halpern et al. (2008) support Zeisel's visitor-centered approach. They found that the aesthetic preferences of individuals with Alzheimer's disease remained stable even when these individuals could not remember ever having viewed the paintings in the study before. In-depth guidelines produced by staff of Visual Understanding in Education (1998) to assist in the selection of images for beginning viewers can be very helpful to designers of a new program. These guidelines consider relevant aspects of the works, including cognitive accessibility, expressive content, narrative, realism, media, and genre. Key recommendations include: (i) ensuring that all participants can easily see the work being discussed (for elderly visitors, this may argue against dark paintings with very small images); (ii) selecting representational rather than abstract art, so that visitors can easily recognize persons and objects; (iii) presenting the works of art in a series, united by some visual elements or themes; and (iv) sequencing the works of art from simpler to complex in terms of number of details, density of content, and ambiguity of meaning.

Time Allocation

Findings and experiences from the current study, as well as from Housen (2001), Ritchhart (2007), Tishman and Palmer (2006), Visual Understanding in Education (1998) and Zeisel (2009), strongly recommend that visitors interact with three to five works of art for approximately twelve to fifteen minutes each for a total of no more than one hour at a time. In order to create a high quality context for visitor engagement and extended discussion, it is more important to spend sufficient time with very few works of art than to have a rushed experience with many.

Size and Constitution of the Group

In order to allow each visitor the opportunity to be in a good position to view the work of art, and ask questions, recount memories, and express opinions at each stop on the tour, only two to six individuals should be included in each group. If the group has four or more visitors in it, having two guides (or one guide and a museum volunteer) is highly recommended, as this will allow one of the guides to facilitate communication as he or she sits or stands among the visitors.

Discussion Routines

In her powerful presentation on aesthetic and art education, Housen (2001: 14) notes the importance of language use in creating an "environment of group discovery," both in the "carefully crafted questions" that focus visitors' attention and in the process of dialogue that "keeps attention focused in a desired way and allows a course of puzzling and construction to unfold." Following Housen, then, it is critical for museum guides to have a communicative routine in mind before the tour begins. Such routines assist the visitor in knowing what to expect of the situation, enabling him or her to speak more freely. Ritchhart (2007: 146) refers to a pattern of questioning used by the Queensland University of Technology Museums Collaborative, a pattern that focuses discussion in the four stages of description, analysis, interpretation, and judgment, and which may be useful with individuals at earlier stages of Alzheimer's disease. Zeisel (2009: 90–97) outlines 11 communication principles, including the use of "simple descriptions and questions" that relate to "something specific in the work." In order to allow for a wider range of possible responses by visitors, it is recommended to begin the tour with questions about each work of art (Housen 2001: 15): "What's going on here?" followed by "What do you see that makes you say that?". Ritchhart (2007: 147) points out that this particular routine—with the addition of a third question: "What more can you find?"—focuses on the "learner's own interpretation and analysis without the addition of information from the tour guide."

As these discussion routines are set in motion within the actual context of a work of art, guides should remain flexible, following the lead of language used by the visitors. If the primary goal of the museum-based activity is to provide an opportunity for those with Alzheimer's disease to engage in a meaningful way both with works of art and with others (and less so on the acquiring of specific knowledge about artists and works of art), then guides should encourage conversation by starting generally and give time for visitors to think and respond to the guide and to each other. If open-ended questions do not result in extended responses by visitors, the guide can then pose a question that focuses group attention on details in the work of art. Such specificity may well prompt discussion of an object, a painting technique, or a story line. It has to be kept in mind, however, that the posing of specific questions limits the type of responses visitors can give and may inhibit changes in topic by visitors that could result in a more energized discussion. On the power of questions to control conversational topics see Ainsworth-Vaughn (1998). According to Ritchhart (2007: 150), it is perhaps most important for museum guides to show "genuine interest in [. . .] ideas and thoughts during the tour" by asking follow-up or clarification questions or adding more details of their own.

In closing, I am hopeful that this study has provided a solid first step in illuminating the contextual relationship between language and Alzheimer's disease within the special context of an art museum, while simultaneously providing a guide to improving everyday lives of people living with the disease through interesting activities that promote extensive talk. When used by sensitive tour guides, works of art that serve as physical anchors in the here and now can spark lively verbal communication among those with Alzheimer's disease. In this process, displays of emotion, knowledge, and control can be encouraged and nurtured—aspects of human communication that are central to the ongoing and vital construction of self-esteem and self-identity.

Notes

I am grateful to Michael Bird and Anneliese Blair, primary investigators of "A Pilot Evaluation of Access to Art Gallery Tours for People with Dementia" for including me in this intriguing and important project and forwarding to me the audio recordings of the museum tours and digital images of the works of art viewed at the National Gallery of Australia in New South Wales, Australia. Bird and Blair are clinical psychologists in the Aged Care Evaluation Unit at the Greater Southern Area Health Service in Queanbeyan, New South Wales.

[1] In fact, according to Leinhardt and Knutson (2004: 81), their investigation of conversations among non-guided visitors to museums represents the only study

that deals exclusively with discursive practices of museums in general, although they explicitly exclude guided tours from their data set.

[2] Transcription conventions:

XXX	unintelligible
/phrase/	uncertain transcription
[	overlapping speech
{ }	details regarding voice quality, nonverbal noise
{choral}	several people talking at once
=	continuation on later line, or from previous line
-	cut-off speech, or false starts

[3] Permission was not granted by the copyright holder of this painting for the reproduction of its image in this chapter. Interested readers can view the painting at: http://cs.nga.gov.au/Detail.cfm?IRN=109694

[4] Zeisel (2009: 103–04) provides details regarding a "do-it-yourself" program for friends and family of an individual with Alzheimer's disease who would like to set up a personal program that involves works of art.

References

Abelson, R. P. (1963). Computer simulation of 'hot cognition'. In S. Tomkins & S. Messick (eds), *Computer Simulation and Personality: Frontier of Psychological Theory*, 277–98. New York: Wiley.

Ainsworth-Vaughn, Nancy. (1998). *Claiming Power in Doctor-patient Talk.* Oxford: Oxford University Press.

Appell, J., A. Kertesz & M. Fisman. (1982). A study of language functioning in Alzheimer patients. *Brain and Language* 17. 73–91.

Bayles, K. A. & A. Kaszniak. (1987). *Communication and Cognition in Normal Aging and Dementia.* Boston, MA: Little, Brown and Company.

Blakemore, Bill. (2006). Art awakens Alzheimer's patients' minds. *ABC News*, 2 July. http://abcnews.go.com/WNT/Health/story?id=2146253&page=1 (last accessed 15 September 2010).

Chafe, Wallace. (1994). *Discourse, Consciousness and Time: The Flow and Displacement of Conscious Experience in Speaking and Writing.* Chicago, IL: University of Chicago Press.

Cohen, A. & C. Eisdorfer. (1986). *The Loss of Self.* New York: Norton.

Davis, Boyd H. (ed.). (2005). *Alzheimer Talk, Text and Context: Enhancing Communication.* New York: Palgrave Macmillan.

De Fina, Anna, Deborah Schiffrin & Michael Bamberg (eds). (2006). *Discourse and Identity.* Cambridge, MA: Cambridge University Press.

Erickson, Frederick. n.d. Hot cognition in a heated argument: Work in progress on the interactional situation of learning. Unpublished manuscript, University of California, Los Angeles.

Goffman, Erving. (1974). *Frame Analysis: An Essay on the Organization of Experience.* New York: Harper & Row.

Grishin, Sasha. (2002). Latin American Grand Final. In Anne Gray (ed.), *Australian Art in the National Gallery of Australia, 280.* Canberra: National Gallery of Australia.

Halpern, Andrea R., Jenny Ly, Seth Elkin-Frankston & Margaret G. O'Connor. (2008). 'I know what I like': Stability of aesthetic preference in Alzheimer's patients. *Brain and Cognition* 66. 65–72.

Hamilton, Heidi E. (1994a). *Conversations with an Alzheimer's Patient: An Interactional Sociolinguistic Study.* Cambridge: Cambridge University Press.

—(1994b). Requests for clarification as evidence of pragmatic comprehension difficulty: The case of Alzheimer's disease. In Ronald L. Bloom, Loraine K. Obler, Susan De Santi & Jonathan S. Ehrlich (eds), *Discourse Analysis and Applications: Studies in Adult Clinical Populations,* 185–200. New York: Lawrence Erlbaum, Inc.

—(1996). Intratextuality, intertextuality, and the construction of identity as patient in Alzheimer's disease. *Text* 16 (1). 61–90.

—(2000). Dealing with declining health in old age: Identity construction in the Oppen Family letter exchange. In: Joy Peyton, Peg Griffin, Walt Wolfram & Ralph Fasold (eds), *Language in Action: New Studies of Language in Society,* 599–610. Cresskill, NJ: Hampton Press.

—(2008). Narrative as snapshot: Glimpses into the past in Alzheimer's discourse. *Narrative Inquiry* 18(1). 53–82.

Heritage, John. (1997). Conversation analysis and institutional talk: Analyzing data. In David Silverman (ed.), *Qualitative Research: Theory, Method and Practice,* 222–45. London: Sage.

Housen, Abigail. (2001). *Eye of the Beholder: Research, Theory and Practice.* Paper presented at the Aesthetic and Art Education: A Transdisciplinary Approach Conference, Lisbon, Portugal, 27–29 September 1999.

Housen, Abigail & Philip Yenawine. (2001). Guide to museum visits. www.vtshome.org/system/resources/0000/0022/guide_to_museum_visits.pdf (last accessed 15 September 2010).

Kempler, Daniel. (1984). *Syntactic and Symbolic Abilities in Alzheimer's Disease.* Unpublished Ph.D. dissertation, University of California, Los Angeles.

Kennedy, Randy. (2005). The Pablo Picasso Alzheimer's therapy. The *New York Times,* 30 October. www.nytimes.com/2005/10/30/arts/design/30kenn.html (last accessed 15 September 2010).

Kitwood, Tom. (1988). The technical, the personal, and the framing of dementia. *Social Behaviour* 3. 161–79.

Lazarus, R. S. & C. A. Smith. (1988). Knowledge and appraisal in the cognition-emotion relationship. *Cognition and Emotion* 2(4). 281–300.

Leinhardt, Gaea & K. Crowley. (2002). Objects of learning, objects of talk: Changing minds in museums. In S. Paris (ed.), *Multiple Perspectives on Object-centered Learning,* 301–24. Mahwah, NJ: Lawrence Erlbaum Associates.

Leinhardt, Gaea & Karen Knutson. (2004). *Listening in on Museum Conversations.* Walnut Creek, CA: Altamira Press.

MacPherson, Sarah, Michael Bird, Katrina Anderson, Terri Davis & Annaliese Blair. (2009). An art gallery access programme for people with dementia: 'You do it for the moment'. *Aging & Mental Health* 13(5). 744–52.

Obler, Loraine K. (1981). Review of 'Le langage des dements' by Luce Irigaray. *Brain and Language* 12. 375–86.

Perkins, David. (2003). *Making Thinking Visible.* New Horizons. www.newhorizons.org/strategies/thinking.perkins.htm (accessed 1 June 2010).

Ramanathan, Vai. (1997). *Alzheimer Discourse: Some Sociolinguistic Dimensions.* Mahwah, NJ: Erlbaum.

Ritchhart, Ron. (2007). Cultivating a culture of thinking in museums. *Journal of Museum Education* 32(2). 137–54.

Sabat, Steven. (2001). *The Experience of Alzheimer's Disease: Life Through a Tangled Veil.* Oxford: Blackwell.

Sabat, Steven & Rom Harré. (1992). The construction and deconstruction of self in Alzheimer's disease. *Ageing and Society* 12. 443–61.

Sacks, H., E. A. Schegloff & G. Jefferson. (1974). A simplest systematics for the organization of turn-taking for conversation. *Language* 50. 696–735.

Schegloff, E. A. & H. Sacks. (1973). Opening up closings. *Semiotica* 8. 289–327.

Schiffrin, Deborah. (1996). Narrative as self-portrait: The sociolinguistic construction of identity. *Language in Society* 25(2). 167–203.

Shenk, Dana. (2005). There was an old woman: Maintenance of identity by people with Alzheimer's dementia. In Boyd H. Davis (ed.), *Alzheimer Talk, Text and Context,* 3–17. New York: Palgrave Macmillan.

Tishman, Shari & Patricia Palmer. (2006). *Artful Thinking: Stronger Thinking and Learning Through the Power of Art.* Final report submitted to Traverse City Area Public Schools by the President and Fellows of Harvard College, Project Zero, Harvard Graduate School of Education, Cambridge. www.pz.harvard.edu/Research/ArtfulThinkingFinalReport.pdf (last accessed 15 September 2010).

Visual Understanding in Education. (1998). *Guidelines for Image Selection for Beginning Viewers.* www.vtshome.org/system/resources/0000/0211/Guidelines_for_Image_Selection.pdf (last accessed 15 September 2010).

Zeisel, John. (2009). *I'm Still Here: A Breakthrough Approach to Understanding Someone Living with Alzheimer's.* New York: Penguin Group.

Chapter 10

Using Narrative Arts to Foster Personhood in Dementia

Ellen B. Ryan and Lori Schindel Martin

Introduction

The cognitive losses in dementia and the excess disability associated with the label of dementia threaten personal identity and sense of self (Fontana and Smith 1989). Opportunities for communication are especially constrained for individuals with dementia who reside in assisted living or long-term care facilities (MacDonald, 2006). The construction, telling or writing, and sharing of stories serve to promote connections between the person living with dementia and others, thereby fostering personhood.

This chapter will explain the use of narrative arts in the promotion of personhood in dementia care. It addresses the use of narrative arts such as storytelling, life writing, memory boxes, and collaborative poetry, and provides case examples. The clinical implications of narrative arts for the care of persons with dementia as well as staff development needs are also discussed. We begin with a description of the Canadian context for research concerning older adults with dementia.

Aging, Dementia, and Caregiving in Canada

Canada's population of older people is growing, increasing from 11% of the total population in 1987 to 13% in 2007. By 2056, it is anticipated that the number of people over the age of 65 years will further increase to 27% of the total population. It is forecasted that the population segment that will experience the most growth will be older people over the age of 80 years. This group is predicted to increase from 3% of the total population in 2007 to 10% by 2056 (Statistics Canada 2008). Given that age is considered to be the number one risk factor for Alzheimer's disease and related dementias (ADRD), the aging of Canada's population will have direct consequences on the number of people living with these illnesses. The incidence of ADRD in Canada was 103,700 new cases per year by 2008. The prevalence of ADRD in Canada was 480,600 people (1.5% of the total population) in 2008. This is expected to rise to 1,125,184 or 2.8% of Canada's total population by 2038 (ASC 2010).

The economic costs associated with ADRD are considerable. It is estimated that the cumulative incidence of dementia will be more than 5.5 million people by 2038, with an associated economic cost of C$872 billion. While individuals with dementia in the early to moderate stages of the illness will most likely be cared for at home, most persons in the later stages of the illness will require some type of facility-based care. In 2008, 45% of Canadians with dementia over the age of 65 years were being cared for in long-term care homes. It is anticipated that the demand for long-term care beds will increase but there will most likely be a shortfall (ASC 2010).

Clearly, the burden associated with care that is and will be needed for older people with ADRD demands attention to the development and testing of creative, useful interventions. Narrative arts offer important approaches to enhance the care for such individuals, particularly those in mid to late stages of the disease process who are living in facility-based care.

Personhood in Dementia Care

Within the biomedical paradigm, personhood is frequently presented as dependent on cognition. Until recent times, the predominant health care discourse focused on understanding the deterioration or "de-selfing" of the person with dementia (Fontana and Smith 1989). This negative discourse was challenged by Kitwood (1990, 1993, 1997), who argued that—instead of focusing on intellect, cognitive capacity, and autonomy—personhood should be based on feelings and the ability to live in relationships. He conceptualized personhood as a status that is granted upon one person by others within the context of their social interactions. Personhood is recognized and validated through the relationship-centered aspects of conversation and communication through engagement, insightful listening, acknowledgement of emotions, sharing ideas, reflection, and demonstrating acceptance. Kitwood believed that personhood can be maintained for individuals living with dementia by enabling choice, the use of remaining abilities, and expression of feelings.

Sabat and Harré (1992) have also argued that the excess disability created by others around dementia threatens the self as much as the disease itself. Through detailed presentation of personhood-oriented conversations, Sabat (2001) has shown that people with moderate to severe dementia can connect with a conversational partner and overcome the loss of self-worth associated with their typical treatment. Furthermore, he has shown how inappropriate behaviors, usually taken as symptoms of pathology, are often strategies for coping with boredom, frustration, and isolation (see also Hughes et al. 2006). Through the work of Kitwood, Sabat, and others, an emergent key theme is that efforts to find the person behind the dementia repay the caregiver with reciprocity, creativity, and humor.

Placement in long-term care homes can have a negative impact on both the person with dementia and their family caregivers. Emotional distress and depression are common during the post-institutionalization transition period (Paun and Farran 2006). According to Brooker (2007), formal caregivers can promote person-centered care of persons with dementia by regularly asking clients and families for their preferences, consent, opinions, and thinking about decisions from the residents' point of view, as well as being attentive to and recognizing physical needs, and analyzing challenging behavior to understand underlying reasons for it. Developing these habits can prevent formal caregivers from attaching stereotypical meanings to behavior by bringing the person's unique personhood into clear view.

Creating a supportive social environment is also a means of getting to know residents' personal characteristics. Brooker (2007) encourages the inclusion of residents with dementia in conversation, that is, treating them with respect, warmth, and acceptance, taking their fears seriously, helping them be active in their care, and keeping them in contact with the community. Attentiveness to social needs and encouraging involvement in these ways can help to continuously remind staff of residents' personal identities. While Brooker's recommendations are reasonable, it is important for professional caregivers to identify specific interventions that help build and maintain a rich social environment by taking the residents' personal identities into full account. Narrative art forms create ideal contexts within which person-centered conversations can take place.

Narrative Arts in Dementia Care

Older adults with dementia usually experience an impoverished social environment unless conscious, deliberate opportunities to engage in meaningful conversation are provided (Hopper et al. 2007). Older adults with cognitive impairment experience decline in various aspects of language function, including narrative discourse. Narrative discourse involves the oral representation of a significant, meaningful event or series of events in a person's life. Narrative discourse capacity is impaired in ADRD as a result of reduced access to vocabulary and to poorer topic management skills (Davis 2005). However, persons with ADRD can often produce socially ritualized aspects of conversation, particularly when facilitated by other people who are familiar with the individual's typical communicative strategies such as pitch, rate, intensity, movements, facial expression, and gestures (Moss et al. 2002). It is increasingly apparent that arts-based therapies such as visual art, music, drama, poetry, horticulture, dance, and storytelling can be important vehicles for patients to express their thoughts, emotions, and ideas in symbolic fashion. It is the process of creation, not the product that remains the focus of such intervention (Lamb 2009).

In particular, the sharing of stories is a medium through which people who are ill can transcend their experience of illness so that their humanness is affirmed (Cangelosi and Sorrell 2008; Frank 1995; Mitty 2010; Scott and DeBrew 2009). In the case of an older person with advanced dementia, the storyteller is often a family member or formal caregiver, who, by telling the story, bears witness to the survival of the person's fundamental spirit. By preserving and re-telling the older person's favorite stories, the caregiver becomes a guide and witness. In this context, storytelling builds and maintains personal identity, thus serving a transformative purpose (Mitty 2010). Persons in various stages of dementia can succeed in telling episodes from their lives or in writing life stories within a facilitating environment. The goal of narrative arts in dementia care is to provide just the right assistance so that the person can express their message—the voice is their own. The narrative arts we address here include storytelling, facilitated writing, and narrative thematic conversation.

Storytelling to Connect

Storytelling reconstructs personal identity through active exchange with the listener. Thus, the story serves as a medium to sustain the self while at the same time communicating information about the self with others. The storyteller can choose to select life events that will be shared, and some details may become embellished or be eliminated over time. The telling and retelling of the story will continue to change and shape personal identity as the plot ebbs and flows (Holstein and Gubrium 2000). Stories inform us who we were, who we are now, and who we could be if all things were possible. Stories also help all people, including those living with dementia, to make sense of what has happened, what is presently happening, and what they fear might happen to them in an unknown future (Somers 1994). Past, present, and future become linked and understood through the chronology of events presented in life stories. Personal identity is reinforced as the story of the self changes (Rasmussen 1995). By telling and retelling personal stories, older adults engage others in conversation that reinforces and shapes their identity and their position within the internal and external world.

Through a series of case studies, we have come to understand how conversation based on narrative art forms between persons with dementia and their formal caregivers can lead to the building and remodeling of a personal story to fit shifting circumstances. We have discovered how building the story together, then telling, writing, and retelling the story leads to conversation and relationship, and how relationship and story lead to a sense of belonging and reclaimed identity. While the stories are important in themselves, they also have direct application to clinical situations, thus enhancing professional caregiving.

Life Story Dictation

Personal storytelling can be used by caregivers to help the person reconnect with life moments and family members of great importance (Ryan, Schindel Martin and Beamer 2005). As one example, life story dictation was used in clinical practice to address an older client's repetitive yearning for her long-dead mother—creating, telling, and rereading the story of her mother acknowledged and satisfied the deep need underneath this seemingly impossible request.

Case Example

Mrs. Hazel Broadfoote (pseudonym) was a 98-year-old resident of a long-term care facility situated in Central Ontario. Mrs. B grew up on a rural dairy farm that had been owned by her family for many generations. The family were United Empire Loyalists who originally came to Canada from rural Pennsylvania just prior to the revolutionary war in the United States. Mrs. B married at the age of 16 to a second cousin who took over her parents' farm. Together they raised five children. Despite hard times during the depression, Mrs. B was proud that they always served nutritious food at the table, and were able to provide free lodging to the schoolteacher who taught at the local one-room school house. Mr. and Mrs. B retired in 1968 and moved to town where they became actively involved in church life. Mr. B died in 1982, and Mrs. B continued to live in their home until her daughters noticed that she was beginning to have trouble cooking and preparing food. She lost approximately 30 pounds over the space of 3 months. She was admitted to a long-term care facility after a fire broke out in the kitchen. Mrs. B's daughters all live nearby and take turns visiting her. Mrs. B frequently interprets her surroundings as the bus station. She frequently asks passersby for a "nickel" for the bus so she can get to the farmer's market to help her mother. In fact, her major preoccupation most days is to roam the hallways and dining room of the long-term care home looking for her mother. She talks of needing to get the cows in for milking, or hoping her mother isn't angry because she thinks the cows have been forgotten in the pasture. Sometimes she becomes agitated because she needs to leave to get the cows in before her mother returns from market.

The health care team worked directly with Mrs. B to record many details with respect to her mother, family, and farm life. These details have been written into the form of a story in which Mrs. B is cast as the main "character" as a young child. Copies of the story were recorded in large print text, and when Mrs. B became agitated, the formal caregivers would engage her in the following conversation:

(1) Conversation between MRS. B and TEAM MEMBER

MRS. B:	"Have you got a nickel for the bus? I have to take the milk to market. My mother is expecting me. Has she been asking for me?"
TEAM MEMBER:	"Hello Mrs. B. Thank you for stopping by. You are very thoughtful to be asking about your mother."
MRS. B:	"Yes, my mother relies on me."
TEAM MEMBER:	"Yes, you are very reliable. I haven't met your mother, but you've told me many stories about her."
MRS. B:	"Yes, my mother is a very good woman. She is always there to help others, and I want to help her too."
TEAM MEMBER:	"Yes, you've told me that your mother was an excellent cook, and a very important member of the church you attended when you were a little girl. The church was on Concession 17. Your farm was on Concession 19, just off the Arkell Road."
MRS. B:	"Why yes, have you visited us there?"
TEAM MEMBER:	"No, I haven't, but I feel like I have. You've told me a lot about it." [The team member then reaches for the story, copies of which are always kept at the team station, and begins to read excerpts from the written stories by starting with] "In fact, here are some stories you've told me of the farm that you grew up on . . ."

Mrs. B would listen to these stories and provide additional details such as "There was an iron gate that led to the front garden. Mother wouldn't let us swing on the gate. We always did anyway. One day I fell off the gate and mother said that was why I have flat feet." The additional details were added to the story over time so that it included moments of significance from life events and thus had more meaning for Mrs. B. Layering in additional details as she told more stories allowed us to give back information that led her to feel deeply "understood." While this process was not always helpful, for example, if Mrs. B was physically ill, the storytelling approach was very effective for the majority of episodes. Indeed, Mrs. B's response to the storytelling was used as a clinical predictor of the etiology of her agitation. If she did not respond positively to the story, it was hypothesized that her agitation might be the result of a medical problem, such as a urinary tract infection; therefore, treatment needs could be identified.

Life storytelling is a tool through which professional and family caregivers can help the older person with dementia make sense of the present moment. Without the story, reassurance will not be as meaningful or effective. The story grounds reassurance in the context of familiar, concrete life events through things only a real friend would know about and share back and forth on a regular basis. This helps staff to have very specific life events to retell to the resident, thus avoiding general platitudes such as "don't worry, you're okay" that only serve to patronize and frustrate the individual. In this case example, life storytelling brought Mrs. Broadfoote's mother "back to her," not in person but, rather more importantly, in essence.

Conversational Remembering Boxes

The Conversational Remembering Box represents another strategy we have developed to engage persons with dementia and promote personhood-preserving strategies in conversation and storytelling (Hagens et al. 2003). At the early stage of dementia, individuals can be encouraged to prepare their own Remembering Box which they can use when conversation becomes difficult. At the moderate or late/moderate stages of dementia, family and staff can initiate the preparation of a Remembering Box, with pictures, objects, audio/video tapes, and writings. The box itself can be meaningful, such as a nostalgic hatbox from the 1940s or a man's longtime fishing tackle box. Remembering Boxes have included personal and family photos, pictures, and information related to homes and travels (saved or from the Internet), religious items, medals, or award certificates, hobby materials such as fabric for a quilter, favorite music and movies, grandchildren's letters or drawings, and ancient or recent letters.

In our experience, written (or taped) records of individuals telling their stories in their own words are very important for the Remembering Box. Individuals able to read aloud often begin adding to their stories when reading their own words (the use of larger fonts can often help). Those unable to read are often induced to continue their story by hearing their own favorite expressions, their own way of telling that story (see also Davis and Smith, this volume). The Remembering Box is intended to grow and change over time as new items are brought for inclusion. Most importantly, a journal is included in the box so that visitors/staff can write down new stories and additional details offered by the individual. The best of these are later typed for inclusion in the Box.

The Remembering Box can be used by family or staff to engage the individual in conversation. Again, the critical element here is that a memory box is much more than the opportunity to present familiar objects. Rather, it is a process whereby elements of the self are introduced to reinforce personhood. This resource helps family members move away from short-term memory questions, which are so problematic for the person with dementia, and toward conversational topics where the person with dementia can often participate "richly" and become "more like themselves." Staff responses in Hagens et al. (2003) showed that long-term care residents wanted visitors in the room to look into the box (even if not remembering why) and that they were sometimes able to take control of the conversation as they remembered. This resource can be especially useful when long-term care staff have just a few minutes to talk or when the resident is agitated in the middle of the night. Finally, creating a Remembering Box is an excellent activity for family to carry out with loved ones moving into long-term care.

Basting in her (2009) book on dementia demonstrates the deep desire of both individuals with dementia and their families to connect in the present and for the purposes of creating a legacy: the Remembering Box, especially the written stories in the person's own words, connect in the present and also serve as a valuable legacy for family. Furthermore, Basting (2007) reports that individuals with dementia and their families have been eager to participate in the StoryCorps Memory Loss Initiative. In this initiative, a family member or friend is guided in deep listening and the asking of appropriate questions to elicit stories from the person with dementia in an audio recording booth. The recorded stories, Basting showed, become a magnificent mutual family accomplishment as well as a valued contribution to a legacy. Such audio (or video) recordings would fit very well in the person's Remembering Box.

Case Example

Mrs. Verna Stemple was a 79-year-old resident in a long-term care facility who had made her living in Paris as a seamstress. She had worked for a couture fashion house for many years. She came to Canada just before WWII broke out in Europe. She was called upon by many famous people in the Toronto arts community to design and sew replica ball gowns and dresses for parties during the 1950s and 1960s. For example, they would bring her photos of Jacqueline Kennedy published in *Look* magazine and ask her to design something similar to wear during the holiday season. Mrs. S enjoyed some degree of celebrity during this time. After admission to the long-term care facility she became quite certain that no one knew who she was, not as the mother of her children, and wife of her husband, but as the very famous seamstress who enjoyed considerable success. Her family brought in her seamstress measuring tape, her thimbles, her patterns, sketches, and photos, and all were placed in a Remembering Box. Both professional staff and family members used the items from the box regularly. Mrs. S was particularly fond of looking at the photograph of her youngest daughter in the wedding gown that Mrs. S had designed and sewn for her. Although she did not recognize her daughter in person, she absolutely knew who the person in the picture was, and this photo in the Remembering Box served as the bridge through which mother and daughter could connect in the past/present moment.

Facilitated Writing

Many older adults enjoy putting stories from their lives into written form—through personal journals or letters initially and, for some, then sharing written stories more widely with family or a writing group or through publication of memoirs and autobiographies (Ray 2000). As presented in Ryan (2006), individuals experiencing chronic illness or acquired disability, including dementia, have been drawn to write as a means to reflect systematically on their experiences and threatened sense of self. Finding one's voice through personal writing fosters self-expression, creativity, emotional outlet, problem solving, perspective taking, and memory. For persons whose condition, like dementia, is associated with communication and memory problems, writing one's story offers some specific benefits over telling one's story orally. These specific benefits include: greater control over time, topic, and environment; flexible pace; reliance on others or on technology not visible in the product; less reliance on good memory; no need for hearing or monitoring nonverbal cues (Ryan, Spykerman and Anas 2005; Ryan 2006). Moreover, the ideal reader understands perfectly so there is no need to have a specific interested and empathetic listener immediately at hand.

Memoir Writing

Some individuals with diagnoses of probable Alzheimer's disease have published their memoirs in book or essay form. Basting's (2003) analysis of books by three authors offered numerous insights into dementia, especially about the continuing sense of self. Ryan and colleagues (2009) extended this work by analyzing the published dementia memoirs of nine writers, using the authors' own words to show how these individuals, after being diagnosed with Alzheimer's or related neurological disorders, had reclaimed their identity through their writing roles as creators, chroniclers, teachers, advocates, and social contributors.

Dementia memoirs articulately and compellingly counter the stereotypes of persons with dementia as no longer capable of new learning and as without insight into their losses and strengths. These autobiographical writings each put a distinctive face on dementia and draw attention to the accomplishments possible after such a diagnosis. The metaphoric language characteristic of dementia, as Killick and Allan have shown (2001), emerges especially positively as authors reach for words to describe what is happening to them. The following are a few examples of particularly telling metaphorical language, collected from various memoirs.

> My mind has become a sieve that can only catch and hold certain random things. (Davis 1989: 21)
>
> My long-term memory is left battered; trying to find moments of the past is like fishing with a dull, rusting hook without bait. (DeBaggio 2003: 205)
>
> The unreliability of my memory is as if the printer ink is running low and it sometimes works and sometimes doesn't. (Bryden 2005: 106)
>
> When I first stumbled across Dr. Alzheimer in my brain, he was an occasional nuisance. He would empty a room full of memories here and there, and cause a couple of doors to stick, but I devised strategies to get around his tricks. (Taylor 2007: 65)

Authors describe counter-stereotypical experiences such as learning to use the computer after diagnosis as a way to cope with deteriorating handwriting and as a means of staying in touch with people when going out has become difficult. Under favorable writing conditions, they can recount daily experiences of figuring out how to get something done when they cannot rely on their memory and give reasonable explanations for their otherwise weird behavior. For example, Henderson in his Alzheimer's journal (1998) explains (to his daughter) that he froze on the stairs the day before because his vision was so distorted he could not tell whether the stairs went up or down at a time when his ability to talk had also fled.

Authors with dementia write about how they manage to write a book, giving worthy insights on adaptation to cognitive difficulties and wise use of technical and family help. Most poignantly, they write about how the behavior of others constrains their opportunities to participate in life and realize their potential.

> If we do believe the lie of dementia, that we can't learn new things, remember anything reliably, or find our way around, we are blindfolded to our own potential. We withdraw into helplessness and let our families take over. (Bryden 2005: 143)
>
> I think for a lot of us the feeling of being cheated, or the feeling of being belittled and somehow made jokes of, I think that's one thing that is among the worst things about Alzheimer's. (Henderson 1998: 37)
>
> Watch my face for hints that I do not understand. Sometimes I don't speak, but my nonverbals shout [. . .] It is not so much what people say; it is how they say it. It is their body language. (Taylor 2007: 153, 189)

For these authors, writing first for themselves and then for publication has been the way out of the narrow confines of otherwise low expectations for persons with dementia. They experience a rich sense of contribution as they share, teach, and advocate:

> While I am still able to communicate, I want to share this incredible journey into Alzheimer's disease. (Davis 1989: 20)
>
> This book is a chronicle of my battle with Alzheimer's. It is a plain-language, 'as it happened' chronicle which I pray will assist others like me who are dealing with this perplexing problem, and their families [. . .] I feel I'm a pebble in a rapid brook. I hope this little pebble can send out ripples upon ripples, in an ever widening circle, until the ripples eventually lap up on a shore where someone like me is stranded and feeling alone. (McGowin 1993: viii, 118).
>
> I am working today, tapping at this keyboard with little time left, in an attempt to understand who I was and what is left. (DeBaggio 2003: 204)

> I choose a new identity as a survivor. I want to learn to dance with dementia. I want to live positively each day, in a vital relationship of trust with my care-partners alongside me. By [...] focusing on my spirit rather than my mind, I can be free of fear of loss of self, and in so doing can also help you to lose your fear that you are losing me. (Bryden 2005: 170)
>
> Why not see us as a source of answers to our problems, rather than as a source of problems to which our caregivers need answers. We, too, want to be proactive when dealing with our symptoms, not just reactive to our problems! (Taylor 2007: 68)

The authority of writers with dementia cannot be denied. These voices offer words to other persons with dementia who no longer have the words and can also inspire them to try writing. Beyond the early stages, writing is most likely if care partners are available to facilitate the process with highly visible markers, computers with large simple fonts, dictation opportunities, and timely encouragement to write when they are particularly lucid. This type of assistance, as well as help in editing, is frequently mentioned by the writers of the published memoirs. For reasons mentioned earlier, persons with dementia can often express themselves better in writing or in dictation than in conversation. Thus, writing provides opportunity for self-mastery, an element essential for the strengthening of personhood.

Facilitated Poetry

Hagens and colleagues (2003, 2006) describe the process of facilitating poetry with small groups of residents with varying levels of cognitive impairment. A facilitator records all the phrases of participants, rereading them throughout the group session, and rearranging them into poetry for the group's response. The process extends the traditional group reminiscence by paying more attention to the specific words of each individual (recording them on an easel for all the group to see and hear), by repeatedly bringing the group back to the theme for the day so that a product can be achieved, by using the participants' own words to nudge them to contribute further, and by creating a product to share outside the group over time.

The creation of poetry also takes advantage of the metaphoric language of dementia (Killick and Allan 2001; Killick 2003). Moreover, the gaps and topic jumps of Alzheimer's discourse can energize a poem, whereas it is often frustrating and confusing in oral or written storytelling. Moreover, a poem with tangentially related phrases from different individuals can work, whereas a joint story would require much more facilitation by the leader.

The group poem presented here—"On Seeing Red"—includes many shifts of subtopic, but all relate to the color theme. Although some of the phrases are generic, some are very specific. Often family members can read the large print framed poem in a resident's room and recognize their loved one's contribution. For example, one husband was astounded and touched to learn that his wife (who had not communicated orally with him for some time) actually remembered his giving her roses at Christmas (only in the early years before life got so busy). Sharing the poems with family and with staff is key, so that each understands that the person remains.

On Seeing Red

Red
Wash it separately.
They called me carrots...
I always wished
my hair was a different colour.
Kids made fun of us...about 1914 it was...
used to make me
all knuckles and teeth.
Made me see red!
I gave her the hardest kiss she ever had.
The colouring does everything.
Makes you smile a smile,
makes you feel good.

Red roses remind me
of someone I love.
Flowers remind me of death and sickness.
When you feel it, you feel it,
when someone you love passes away.

My husband
always gave me
red roses at Christmas.
I think
we did everything
together.
Always had flowers in the house.
I like
every red I see.

(Quoted in Hagens et al. 2006: 109)

These "reminisce and write" activities can be used with one person at a time—for example, to create a life story in the person's own words so that staff can more readily relate personally. The second poem presented here—"Shani's Brushing"—was facilitated by a researcher working with a cognitively intact resident, called Thelma T., and a resident with dementia, called Lily P., who had been a poet. The three met over approximately 20 sessions, with Lily not recognizing Thelma's face or name. Near the end, they learned that Lily did remember Thelma as the lady with the cat.

Most of the poems facilitated with persons with dementia emphasize long-term memory—either semantic memory, verbal expressions, or long ago episodes. This poem demonstrates that a person with moderate dementia, who has great difficulty with conversation and current memory, can be very sensitive to the present and to relationships.

Shani's Brushing

I can't get over that cat helping her do the job.

Now look, he's licking the hand that fixed him.

Look at him,
he's behaving so beautifully.
He's a darling.

He loves that doesn't he?
She loves it too,

but the cat loves it more.
He could get lost,
and wouldn't know where to come back to.
But then again,
he has no reason to leave.

We're talking about a white cat today.
His name is Shani.

(Excerpt, quoted in Hagens et al. 2006: 137)

Creating personal poetry with a facilitator and sharing the poems with a group as well as family and staff provides the opportunity for aspects of the vulnerable "self" in dementia to be expressed, acknowledged, and celebrated. The written words create contexts for ongoing conversations, in which understanding becomes possible at a feeling, imagery level less linked to the losses of dementia than typical conversation.

Narrative Thematic Conversation

For professional caregivers and families of people with dementia it is often difficult to identify and implement strategies that promote and sustain personhood. Storytelling, life writing, and Remembering Boxes are all such strategies. Narrative Thematic Conversation (Schindel Martin, 2007, 2011), an innovative form of narrative arts, is another strategy that can help develop connectedness between the person with dementia and both professional and family caregivers. The construction of the narrative can take the form of a poem, a story, or a visual art piece. The process involves deep listening and recognition of the person. The art products both connect in the moment and provide a narrative record for the resident. The narrative record can then be used as a medium to strengthen the quality of the continuous relationship between the person with dementia and both families and formal caregivers. It is important to recognize that narrative arts cannot be useful in dementia care if they are only displayed as static images. The poem, picture, or story cannot simply be framed and mounted as an object. Rather, the art form becomes a tool that is used to guide conversation so that interactions occurring in the present moment are grounded in tangible meanings from the past.

A case study will be used to illustrate how one example of the narrative arts, a collage, can be utilized as a continuous link between professional care staff, family members, and the person with dementia.

Case Example

Mr. Jimmy Jacobs (pseudonym) was an 83-year-old resident of a long-term care facility situated in a metropolitan area of Central Ontario. Mr. J was born in rural Nova Scotia, a maritime province in Canada. He had begun his working life as a member of the rural constabulary force, but experienced a difficult case involving the investigation of the abuse and subsequent murder of an infant during his rookie year. The case traumatized him to the degree that he suffered symptoms of what we would now diagnose as significant posttraumatic stress disorder (PTSD). Immediately after this traumatic event, Mr. J moved west to Ontario where he worked hard as the sole proprietor of a small, independent used car dealership. He married and divorced three times, twice to his first wife, all within the space of 10 years. He had no long-term relationship after his third divorce. He had one daughter, from whom he was estranged for the better part of 30 years. He spent a lot of his personal time perfecting his considerable skills as a guitarist. He became the lead guitarist in a small country band that enjoyed some success on the local bar circuit. His support network consisted solely of his bandmates. Just prior to admission in the long-term care facility he experienced a one-sided stroke. Consequently, he has no voluntary movement in the left side of his body. His left shoulder was subluxed, and thus would cause him considerable pain and discomfort, particularly during any personal care such as bathing. His agitation was such that during any attempts at personal care he would shout loud profanities at his caregivers. He would also engage in the same behavior with his daughter, with whom he had reestablished a tentative relationship just prior to his stroke.

The care plan for Mr. J was well developed, ensuring pain control for his subluxed shoulder and the neuropathic pain he was experiencing in the left side of his body subsequent to the stroke. It became apparent to the health care team, however, that something at the core of Mr. J's experience was not being acknowledged or "cared for" to the degree that was necessary to establish a therapeutic relationship. Despite good pain control, his agitated behavior continued. The health care team met and decided that it seemed necessary to acknowledge Mr. J as a person in very concrete ways before and during personal care. He seemed to interpret any attempts at personal care as attempts to objectify him. The health care team interviewed some of the members of his band who were continuing to visit him. Based on the personal history and clinical information, we then developed a long list of his personality characteristics, his stories, his hobbies, his life choices that might help us "give back" to him who he saw himself to be. The health care team also interviewed his daughter to determine her memories of Mr. J as a father during his early adult life. These details were then translated to props, pictures, and typed phrases in large print. The members of the health care team who worked with Mr. J to provide direct care, such as bathing, then approached Mr. J and invited him to work with them to develop a collage that represented important aspects of his life. Mr. J was immediately intrigued, and became very engaged in developing the collage. While his left-sided paralysis prevented him from manipulating many of the objects that would make up the collage, he was instrumental in choosing the pictures and their placement in the collage.

The creation of the collage became a top-priority event for Mr. J that he always looked forward to. Rather than shouting at his care providers, he began to speak to them differently, talking about the progress of the collage and additional items that might be added to it. The focus of conversation during bathing became the collage, not uttering threats to the nurses. In this way, the co-creation of this art piece became the medium through which the person with dementia and his formal caregivers could connect and become true partners in care. Mr. J's daughter also became involved in the development of the collage, answering her father's questions about items, and offering her opinions. The collage became the focus of their tentative relationship, and helped to dissolve the tension between them. The collage included pictures of musical instruments, photographs of

Mr. J with his bandmates, pictures of his used car lot, and his other interests such as visiting Canada's lighthouses, fishing, and collecting model automobiles and trains. When the collage was completed, it was presented at a team conference that included Mr. J and his daughter. A photograph of Mr. J holding the collage with two of the team members who helped him construct it was printed in the long-term care facility's newsletter. The picture was added to the bottom of the collage. Mr. J, his daughter, and the health care team agreed that the collage should be framed and displayed at his bedside. The health care team noticed that if they used the collage to initiate any conversations with Mr. J, his displays of anger and agitation were diminished, and for the most part could be averted. In some instances, when Mr. J was having severe pain associated with his stroke-affected left side, the collage would not be effective in reducing agitation. As with the case of Mrs. B, described above, Mr. J's response to the collage was used as a clinical indicator of pain control. Overall, the collage became a focal point that symbolized important events and feelings held by Mr. J about his journey through life. For the health care team the collage also represented the development of a high-quality interpersonal relationship with a client they might otherwise have only seen as challenging. By the time of Mr. J's death, the health care team had developed a deep affection for Mr. J and the collage was presented to his daughter during a memorial service.

Narrative thematic conversation can take many forms. But, as the case study of Mr. J demonstrates, what is important is that the health-care team identify ways that the key elements of the constructed story can be displayed and accessed at a moment's notice for use by both formal care providers and families.

Practical Implications

The communication enhancement model (Ryan et al. 1995) highlights the importance of strategies for caregiving staff to personalize care, so that both recipient and caregiver are empowered. Research that captures the voices of people living with dementia does not show the stereotypical "loss of self" but rather ongoing and creative efforts to cope with dementia as a manageable disability (Beard et al. 2009;

Snyder 2000). The application of narrative arts in conversation and through writing confirms the identity and personhood of people living with dementia, creates connection, and fosters hope.

One of the critical practice implications of narrative art forms and their role in maintaining communication between persons with dementia and their caregivers is educational programs. It is important that all members of the health care team who work with older adults, whether they be professional staff of day programs or long-term care homes, be trained in the use of art forms to promote meaningful conversation. In addition, it is crucial for family caregivers to be educated by resource and support agencies to use narrative art forms to communicate (Charters and Murray 2006). Such programs could include students of professional programs learning ways to express their own knowledge and experience with dementia using art forms. Projects could include building a professional coat of arms and writing a reflective chapter that explains the significance of such for professional practice behaviors. In addition, professional caregivers could be assigned a specific older adult to work with, and design an art piece that would represent the voice of that person and the students' intuitive sense of what their behavior represents. Journaling, poetry, photo-voice as well as creative writing could also be included as a learning tool for professional caregivers. Without policy changes, however, uptake of such interventions is unlikely. Thus, it is vital that health care regulations are extended to identify and support the use of art forms as a practical way to engage the person with dementia in meaningful interactions.

In addition, it is important for professional caregivers to interact with each other so that narrative arts are used by all members of the health care team. It is critical that leisure and recreation therapists are not seen as the only members of the team to take responsibility for designing person-centered art forms that give voice to the personhood of the individual. Because of staffing and human resource restrictions, the very culture of long-term care is set up so that leisure activities are rushed and often a source of stress for both families and residents alike. Thus, all team members can contribute to narrative art forms that are meaningful, yet highly individualized. It is critically important that narrative art forms be understood as very distinct from "art classes" which persons with dementia may be invited to attend. Goyder (2009) explains that, traditionally, older adults with cognitive impairments who live in long-term care facilities only reluctantly engage in set leisure programs because they are coerced and grouped. This is because activities are not designed as an opportunity to "find the self." Rather, they are time-fillers that have no direct bearing on what happens to the older adult at any other time of the day. The products coming out of a program such as this are rarely shared with health care team members, although they might be hung on the wall or seen in an art exhibition. Thus it is important that long-term care funding include the possibility of hiring art therapists who can work not only with older adults with dementia and their families, but also with staff to enhance their skills repertoire in the area of narrative arts. Our vision is that a truly useful enterprise would see all members of the health care team capable of facilitating the development of narrative art forms that would then serve as a consistent basis for care interventions. The art forms are living documents representative of the person's desires, hopes, dreams, and past lives, and directly guide and inform the development of caregiving plans as illustrated in the case of Mr. J described above.

Research has shown that there are benefits that result from narrative art forms that extend far beyond the context of professional caregiving and care interactions. McFadden and McFadden (2011, in press) argue that learning to "walk with people down the road of dementia" can reduce our own fear of aging, death, and loss of memory. They add that persons with dementia can flourish in communities of friendship where all persons—regardless of cognitive status—are valued. Such communities can offer support and connection to all. An insightful formal caregiver who uses narrative art forms to guide practice is essential to the therapeutic relationship. It is our position that without creative art forms to mediate it conversation between professional caregivers and persons with dementia becomes stilted, arcane, and formulaic. Conversations that use art forms as a bridge for connection become more meaningful because they are grounded in what matters to the individual with cognitive impairments, persons who would otherwise be shut off from a deeper experience of the world.

References

ASC (Alzheimer Society of Canada). (2010). *Rising Tide: The Impact of Dementia on Canadian Society.* www.alzheimer.ca/english/rising_tide/rising_tide.htm (accessed 14 April 2010).

Basting, A. D. (2003). Looking back from loss: Views of the self in Alzheimer's disease. *Journal of Aging Studies* 17. 87–99.

—(2007). NPR's StoryCorps initiative helps preserve fading memories. *Aging Today* 28(4). 14–15.

—(2009). *Forget Memory: Creating Better Lives for People with Dementia.* Baltimore, MD: Johns Hopkins University Press.

Beard, R. L., J. Knauss & D. Moyer. (2009). Managing disability and enjoying life: How we reframe dementia through personal narratives. *Journal of Aging Studies* 23. 227–35.

Brooker, D. (2007). *Person-Centred Dementia Care: Making Services Better.* Philadelphia, PA: Jessica Kingsley Publishers.

Bryden, C. (2005). *Dancing with Dementia: My Story of Living Positively with Dementia.* Vancouver: University of British Columbia Press.

Cangelosi, P. & J. Sorrell. (2008). Storytelling as an educational strategy for older adults with chronic illness. *Journal of Psychosocial Nursing* 46(7). 19–22.

Charters, J. & S. Murray. (2006). Design and evaluation of a leisure education program for caregivers of institutionalized care recipients. *Topics in Geriatric Rehabilitation* 22(4). 334–47.

Davis, B. H. (ed.). (2005). *Alzheimer TalkText and Context: Enhancing Communication.* New York: Palgrave Macmillan.

Davis, Robert. (1989). *My Journey into Alzheimer's Disease.* Wheaton, IL: Tyndale House Publishers.

DeBaggio, Thomas. (2003). *When it Gets Dark: An Enlightened Reflection on Life with Alzheimer's.* New York: Free Press.

Fontana, A. & R. Smith. (1989). Alzheimer's disease victims: The unbecoming of self and the normalization of competence. *Sociological Perspectives* 32. 35–46.

Frank, A. (1995). *The Wounded Storyteller: Body, Illness and Ethics.* Chicago, IL: University of Chicago Press.

Goyder, J. (2009). Alzheimer's disease, personhood, and intervention: A perspective. *Alzheimer's Care Today* 10(4). 183–8.

Hagens, C., A. Beaman & E. B. Ryan. (2003). Reminiscing, poetry writing, and remembering boxes: Personhood-centered communication with cognitively impaired older adults. *Activities, Adaptation, and Aging* 27(3/4). 97–112.

Hagens, C., A. Cosentino & E. B. Ryan. (2006). *You Grow out of Winter: Poetry in Long Term Care* (Writing Down Our Years Series, No. 6). Hamilton, Canada: McMaster Centre for Gerontological Studies.

Henderson, Cary Smith. (1998). *Partial View: An Alzheimer's Journal.* Dallas, TX: Southern Methodist University Press.

Holstein, J. & J. Gubrium. (2000). *The Self we Live by: Narrative Identity in a Postmodern World.* Oxford: Oxford University Press.

Hopper, T., S. Cleary, N. Baumack & A. Fragomeni. (2007). Table fellowship: Mealtimes as a context for conversation with individuals who have dementia. *Alzheimer's Care Quarterly* 8(1). 34–42.

Hughes, J., S. Louw & S. Sabat (eds). (2006). *Dementia: Mind, Meaning and the Person.* New York: Oxford University Press.

Killick, J. (2003). Memorializing dementia. *Alzheimer's Care Quarterly* 4. 18–25.

Killick, J. & K. Allan. (2001). *Communication and the Care of People with Dementia.* Buckingham, England: Open University.

Kitwood, T. (1990). The dialectic of dementia: with particular reference to Alzheimer's disease. *Aging and Society* 10. 177–96.

—(1993). Person and process in dementia. *International Journal of Geriatric Psychiatry* 8(7). 541–5.

—(1997). *Dementia Reconsidered: The Person Comes First.* Philadelphia, PA: Open University Press.

Lamb, J. (2009). Creating change: Using the arts to help stop the stigma of mental illness and foster social integration. *Journal of Holistic Nursing* 27(1). 57–65.

MacDonald, K. (2006). Family and staff perceptions of the impact of the long-term care environment on leisure. *Topics in Geriatric Rehabilitation* 22(4). 294–308.

McFadden, S. H. & J. T. McFadden. (2011), in press. *Aging together: Dementia, Friendship, and Flourishing Communities.* Baltimore, MD: Johns Hopkins University Press.

McGowin, D. F. (1993). *Living in the Labyrinth: A Personal Journey Through the Maze of Alzheimer's.* New York: Delacorte Press.

Mitty, E. (2010). Storytelling. *Geriatric Nursing* 31. 58–62.

Moss, S., E. Polignano, C. White, M. Minichiello & T. Sunderland. (2002). Reminiscence group activities and discourse interaction with Alzheimer's disease. *Journal of Gerontological Nursing* 28(8). 36–44.

Paun, O. & C. Farran. (2006). Nursing home placement of persons with Alzheimer's disease. *Alzheimer's Care Quarterly* 7(2). 104–14.

Rasmussen, D. (1995). Rethinking subjectivity: Narrative identity and the self. *Philosophy and Social Criticism* 21(5/6). 159–72.

Ray, R. E. (2000). *Beyond Nostalgia: Aging and Life Story Writing.* Charlottesville, VA: University Press of Virginia.

Ryan, E. B. (2006). Finding a new voice: Writing through health adversity. *Journal of Language and Social Psychology* 25. 423–36.

Ryan, E. B., K. A. Bannister & A. P. Anas. (2009). The dementia narrative: Writing to reclaim social identity. *Journal of Aging Studies* 23. 145–57.

Ryan, E. B., S. D. Meredith, M. J. MacLean & J. B. Orange. (1995). Changing the way we talk with elders: Promoting health using the Communication Enhancement Model. *International Journal of Aging and Human Development* 41(2). 87–105.

Ryan, E. B., L. Schindel Martin & A. Beaman. (2005). Communication strategies to promote spiritual well-being among people with dementia. *Journal of Pastoral Care and Counseling* 59. 43–55.

Ryan, E. B., H. Spykerman & A. Anas. (2005). Writers with dementia: The interplay among reading, writing, and personhood. In B. H. Davis (ed.), *Alzheimer TalkText and Context*, 190–8. New York: Palgrave Macmillan.

Sabat, S. (2001). *The Experience of Alzheimer's Disease: Life Through a Tangled Veil.* Oxford: Blackwell Publishers.

Sabat, S. & R. Harré (1992). The construction and deconstruction of self in Alzheimer's disease. *Aging and Society* 12. 443–61.

Schindel Martin, L. (2007). *Thematic Narrative Conversation.* Paper presented at Festival of International Conferences on Caregiving, Disability, Aging and Technology (FICCDAT). Toronto, Ontario, June 2007.

—(2011, forthcoming). *Narrative Thematic Dictation*: An interpersonal bridging strategy useful in dementia.

Scott, K. & J. K. DeBrew. (2009). Helping older adults find meaning and purpose through storytelling. *Journal of Gerontological Nursing* 35(12). 38–43.

Snyder, L. (2000). *Speaking our Minds: Personal Reflections from Individuals with Alzheimer's.* San Francisco: W. H. Freeman & Co.

Somers, M. 1994. The narrative constitution of identity: a relational and network approach. *Theory and Society* 23. 605–49.

Statistics Canada (2008). *Canada Year Book,* Chapter 28: 'Seniors', 365–74. Cat.:11–402-X.www.statcan.gc.ca/pub/11–402-x/2008000/pdf/seniors-aines-eng.pdf (accessed 14 April 2010).

Taylor, R. (2007). *Alzheimer's From the Inside Out.* Baltimore, MD: Health Professions Press

Notes on Contributors

Peter Backhaus is Assistant Professor at Waseda University, Tokyo. His research interests include sociolinguistics, conversation analysis, and writing and orthography, with special focus on Japanese. He is author of *Linguistic Landscapes* (Multilingual Matters, 2007) and co-editor of a special issue of the *International Journal of the Sociology of Language* (Vol. 200, 2009) on the topic of language and social aging.

Nikolas Coupland is Professor and Director of the Centre for Language and Communication Research at Cardiff University. He was founding co-editor of the *Journal of Sociolinguistics*, and he co-edits the Oxford UP book-series, *Oxford Studies in Sociolinguistics.* He is an elected member of the British Academy of Social Sciences.

Boyd H. Davis is Bonnie E. Cone Professor of Teaching in Applied Linguistics/English and Professor of Gerontology at University of North Carolina–Charlotte. Her areas of interest include sociohistorical linguistics; Alzheimer's speech; narrative, pragmatics and stance; and digital collections of speech. Her most recent books are *Fillers, Pauses and Placeholders* (edited with N. Amiridze and M. Maclagan, Benjamins 2010) and *Alzheimer Talk, Text and Context* (Palgrave 2005). Her 12-year longitudinal collection of conversational interviews with persons with Alzheimer's disease is one cohort in the digital Carolinas Conversations Collection, sponsored by the National Libraries of Medicine.

Hilke Engfer is a PhD Candidate at the University of Southampton, UK. Her dissertation is titled "Dinner with Wilma. On the relation between (inter)subjectivity, memory and emotion management in migrant-in the-family interactions." Her research interests include conversation analysis, social cognition, and interactional psychology.

Annabel Grant has worked as a speech and language therapist for 15 years. She currently teaches in the undergraduate speech language therapy program at Massey University, Auckland. She has a particular interest in acquired language disorders in adults. Her Masters thesis focused on reminiscence conversations between people with dementia and their caregivers.

Heidi E. Hamilton is Professor in the Department of Linguistics, Georgetown University, where she teaches courses in discourse analysis and applications of interactional sociolinguistics. Her research interests focus on issues of language and Alzheimer's disease, language and aging, medical communication, and language learning. Her books include *Conversations with an Alzheimer's Patient* (Cambridge UP, 1994), *Language and Communication in Old Age: Multidisciplinary Perspectives* (Garland, 1999), *Glimmers: A Journey into Alzheimer's Disease* (Riverwood, 2003), *Handbook of Discourse Analysis* (with D. Schiffrin and D. Tannen, Blackwell, 2001), *Linguistics, Language, and the Professions* (with J.W. Alatis and A. Tan, Georgetown UP, 2002) and *Doing Foreign Language* (with C. Crane and A. Bartoshesky, Prentice Hall, 2004). She is currently co-editing the Routledge *Handbook of Language and Health Communication* (with W.S. Chou).

Trine Heinemann is a Post Doctoral researcher at SPIRE/IFKI, University of Southern Denmark. A conversation analyst and linguist by training, her research focuses on the interplay between language and social action, in particular in Danish. She has published a number of articles on interactions between older people and their caretakers in the context of the Danish home help system and has recently started to investigate the organization of interactions in the audiology clinic.

Rosemary Lubinski, Ed.D., is Professor of Communicative Disorders and Science at the University at Buffalo. She is a Fellow of the American Speech-Language and Hearing Association and the author of over 100 chapters and articles on the topic of adult neurogenics and communication problems associated with aging. She has published six texts, including *Dementia and Communication* and *Communication Technologies for the Elderly: Vision, Hearing, and Communication.* Her 4th edition of *Professional Issues in Speech-Language Pathology and Audiology* is in preparation.

Margaret Maclagan is an Associate Professor in Communication Disorders at the University of Canterbury, New Zealand, where she has taught phonetics and linguistics to speech pathology students. Her research interests include sound change over time in New Zealand English and Māori and language change in time over the course of Alzheimer's disease. She is co-author of *New Zealand English: Its Origins and Evolution* (Cambridge UP, 2004) and *New Zealand English* (Edinburgh UP, 2008).

Lori Schindel Martin is Associate Professor and Associate Director of Scholarship, Research and Creativity at the Daphne Cockwell School of Nursing at Ryerson University, Toronto. Her program of research involves applied educational programs related to dementia care. She is the Chair of the Gentle Persuasive Approaches (GPA) Steering Committee, a provincial initiative focusing on the development and evaluation of knowledge translation products designed to enhance the capacity of direct-care staff in the management of responsive/aggressive behavior of older adults with cognitive impairments.

Yoshiko Matsumoto is Associate Professor of East Asian Languages and Cultures, and by courtesy, of Linguistics at Stanford University. Her general research interests are in various aspects of pragmatics, including the role of context in linguistic structure, and sociolinguistic and discourse analyses of language, aging, and gender. She is author of *Noun-Modifying Constructions in Japanese: A Frame Semantic Approach* (Benjamins, 1997), "Dealing with Changes: Humorous Self-Disclosure by Elderly Japanese Women" (*Ageing & Society*, 2009) and editor of *Faces of Aging: The Lived Experiences of the Elderly in Japan* (Stanford UP, 2011).

Ellen Bouchard Ryan is Professor Emeritus at McMaster University, Hamilton, Canada. Working within the Communication Predicament of Aging Model, her research highlights predicaments experienced by vulnerable older adults with cognitive, sensory, and physical impairments and the roles of empowering communication in promoting successful aging with a disability.

Mary K. Smith is Program Coordinator Health and Community Services, Continuing Education, Central Piedmont Community College, Charlotte, North Carolina, where she also coordinates the Allied Health Continuing Education Programs and manages the American Heart Association Training Center. She regularly consults with programs across the region on e-learning and curriculum development, particularly in geriatric care.

Kristine Williams is a Nurse Gerontologist and Associate Professor at the School of Nursing and Associate Scientist in the Gerontology Center at the University of Kansas. She has had a continuous grant funded from the National Institutes of Health to develop and test interventions that improve care for older adults including those with Alzheimer's disease in assisted living and nursing home care settings. Interventions focus on communication to improve care and reduce confusion in frail older adults and have been featured on national news programs. Additional interventions target mood enhancement and cognitive training to extend older adults' independence in activities of daily living.